Fit, Drunk, and Smarter

Timothy J. Marsala

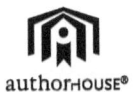

authorHOUSE®

AuthorHouse™
1663 Liberty Drive, Suite 200
Bloomington, IN 47403
www.authorhouse.com
Phone: 1-800-839-8640

www.timothyjmarsala.com
www.fitdrunkandsmarter.com

First published by AuthorHouse 12/26/2007

ISBN: 978-1-4343-2293-7 (sc)

Library of Congress Control Number: 2007905243

Printed in the United States of America
Bloomington, Indiana

This book is printed on acid-free paper.

FIT, DRUNK, & SMARTER!

-TIMOTHY J. MARSALA... FITNESS EXPERT

The college handbook... reveals secrets for avoiding and keeping off the "freshman fifteen," teaches students how to celebrate safer and healthier, and promotes the achievement of academic success!

Fit Drunk and Smarter has been created to empower college-aged students. The author, a Chicago based fitness professional, "trains" young adults on how to remain safe and maintain balance in all aspects of daily life...

Students learn control over alcohol so it won't control them! Everything from physiological and legal ramifications to caloric realities... the truths behind alcohol consumption are revealed. This book does <u>not</u> promote drinking! Instead it provides students with tools such as a B.A.C. (Blood Alcohol Content) chart to prevent the notorious statistics of binging and overdosing on our nation's campuses!

Through valuable dietary recommendations and the signature ten minute workout (10 Minute Tone TM), students are taught how to maintain optimal health while keeping off the "freshman fifteen" for good!

In comparison to many other cultures, many American children have become <u>too</u> gratification oriented, causing unnecessary limitations and even failure. For this reason the book incorporates a heart warming "New Balanced" solution for earning a higher grade point average...while still having fun!

Acknowledgements by: Timothy J. Marsala

Introduction by: Timothy J. Marsala

Foreword by: Dr. Armen S. Kelikian MD
(Professor and Orthopedic Surgeon of Northwestern University and The Chicago Bears)

Chapter 1

Congratulations on Your College Acceptance!
The chapter discusses: 1. Changes students frequently encounter upon transitioning into the college years: Leaving home and abandoning "comfort zones" (internal, social, emotional, and academic) 2. How to recognize and cope with commonly related issues such as homesickness, stress/anxiety, insomnia, and depression 3. Explaining the social polarities between Americans and that of other cultures (Why does *their* academic performance seem to be higher?) 4. Recommending a "New Balanced" attitude to pack in your bags necessary for embracing the stages of higher learning!

Chapter 2

Getting Your Drink On!
Understanding alcohol (and other party enhancing substances)
The chapter will inform the reader of: 1. The physiological effects of alcohol, drugs, and cigarettes upon the body 2. The body's natural inflammatory response to substances (hangovers and our immune system) 3. Legal truths of alcohol and drugs (includes valuable advice from defense attorney Donald Ramsell) 4. The nutritional reality of your cocktails (The caloric values and proofs of hard alcohol, beer, wine, mixers, etc. 5. Which drinks and mixers put the weight on and elevate B.A.C. (Blood Alcohol Content) 6. Safety <u>musts</u> while consuming alcohol/"partying."

Chapter 3

Before the After Party
This chapter discusses: 1. Symptoms of the drinking aftermath! 2. Tips to repair the "hangover" damage: including a. The detoxification process b. The vitality of water and hydration c. Pain relievers d. Purifying food remedies & e. for exercise 3. Pre-partying strategies to avoid a nasty morning after...

Chapter 4

Eating... To become Smarter & Healthier
Your dietary chapter discusses: 1. Foods that hinder and hurt the brain 2. Foods that strengthen the brain by increasing attention span, enhancing memory, alleviating depression, and yes, increasing your I.Q. score... all of which promote a higher GPA. 3. Which foods keep us healthy (anti-oxidants/boosting the immune system) 4. The cleansing and detoxifying foods (fiber/chelation) 5. The importance of acidic vs. alkaline

Chapter 5

Your Meal Plan (Part II)... Eliminate the Freshman 15!
This chapter addresses weight gain in relation to the foods we eat: 1. Are you overweight? Check it out by measuring your B.M.I. (Body Mass Index)

2. What are calories and how many to eat per day? ... 3. The Secrets for achieving Metabolic Balance with your meal plan, The Sugar impact, The truth about carbohydrates, Slimming fiber, How many fat grams per day? And... more water! 3. The importance of breakfast and why it's important to choose foods lower on the Glycemic Index 4. The power of protein 5. What else is keeping the weight on? 6. Eating in social situations 7. More strategies that keep the weight off! 8. How to avoid emotional eating 9. Thinking yourself thin!

Chapter 6

The college lady...
Your chapter discusses social issues during the college years: 1. Dating advice... Where guys' heads are at and where their priorities lay 2. How to tell the good dates from the bad 3. Safety and appropriate conduct 4. What type of women gentlemen are trying to avoid (Cinderella Complex/MRS Degrees) and which ones they're looking to date (the balanced modern lady of today) 6. The effects of alcohol on the female body 7. Stress and Hormones in relation to weight gain 8. Understanding how and why your body may have changed (less tone and the development of cellulite mainly in the hip, thigh and butt regions...)

Chapter 7

The college gentleman...
1. Dating in college: What are the girls looking for, and what they detest about men! 2. Avoiding Peter Pan & 7 common myths many guys believe about girls clarified 3. Safety, & appropriate conduct... i.e. controlling your hormones and frisky libido 4. Male competition: The Pressures to drink each other under the table 5. Safety in Fraternal life/Hazing 6. The negative effects of marijuana and alcohol on the male body (i.e. xenobiotics and testosterone converting into estrogen) 7. How and why guys develop "love handles" and "beer bellies"

Chapter 8

Your New Exercise Lifestyle... Introducing your 10 MINUTE TONE
This chapter teaches students: 1. The importance of exercise 2. Creating the motivation to exercise... extrinsic (which can be limiting or lead to stagnation) vs. beneficial intrinsic motivation 3. The three essentials to instill Motivation and promote an effective workouts (Mental Imagery, Workout buddies, and the Magic of Music all creating momentum) 4. The truth about your fat loss goals/Understanding how we burn fat through exercise (increased

metabolism and through muscle enhancement) 5. How to tone abdominals effectively and why sit ups alone are ineffective for awesome abs/The significance of the "Abdominal Vacuum" 6. The 10 MINUTE TONE TM (Beginning, Moderate and Advanced levels) 7. The Importance of stretching. The 5 most beneficial stretches to incorporate for post work out (Includes advice from expert trainer and Muscle Activation Specialist Ron Greenberg) 8. More effective exercise recommendations...and everyday strategies for burning more calories!

Chapter 9

Case Studies
Laura's story: A nineteen year old second semester freshman implements the dietary, academic, and exercise recommendations (Ten Minute Tone) to 1. Pull up her GPA and 2. Lose the 12 pounds she had accumulated thus so far in her dormitory life. Tommy's story: A 21 year old first semester senior living with friends in an off campus townhouse. He applies the grocery shopping guidelines, heeds Don's legal warnings, and jumpstarts his intramural career along with the Ten Minute Tone to 1. Stay out of trouble, 2. Shed those 8 extra pounds/the beer belly he earned from the first three years of school and to 3. Regain the energy levels he once had in high school!

Footnotes/Works Sited

Glossary of Terms
All of which are relevant to diet, exercise, and legal safety

FIT, DRUNK? AND... SMARTER

The friendly handbook reveals secrets for avoiding the freshman fifteen, how to "celebrate" healthier and safer,...... while enhancing overall academic performance!

Introduction from the Author:

Growing up during the era of the original Incredible Hulk and Charlie's unbelievable Angels, I've always been fascinated by the appearance of the human body. Perhaps my love of WWE Wrestling throughout childhood has led me to desire a strong and ideal physique.

One could also argue that my fascination with fitness could be due to Living a life to the present day cartoon, Fairly Odd Parents. Yeah, I was similar to that little boy with a dreamy mentality of being big and strong conquering anything, especially a baseball.

Coincidentally my name is Timothy, and I did grow up being the youngest and smallest child. Having five older brothers and sisters coupled with extremely hard working and unconditionally supportive parents, left me with the underlying desire to feel and remain physically fit and as staunch as possible.

Anyhow, my love for fitness did carry over into the college years, eventually oiling me up on stage into body building competitions.

Now like any heterosexual male, I absolutely love a beautiful female body. Everything from her naturally toned hips and thighs to a slim waistline. Please understand that this mindset is not necessarily chauvinistic, but is synonymous to admiring an exquisite painting or sunset in the Caribbean.

So I have focused my career as a personal trainer for the past eight years helping people achieve their personal fitness goals. But being "Timmy T." at heart, this book is targeted to a younger (college-aged) audience because I've been there!

The college years can be stressful enough, so I understand the need to blow off steam after mid-terms, and participate in everything that goes along with "Miller Time." Wow, it's amazing how students can stomach the beer-bonging or the quarters games, but it happens. Who knows what causes it, but there's certainly a high that coexists with binge drinking during these years to the point where it's become a bit scary from a statistical standpoint.

Mother Nature will eventually make you grow out of it. But in the meantime, there are ways of taking care of yourself through proper diet, exercise, and a dose of street smarts. Now unless you participate in collegiate sports activities, the college lifestyle can really take a toll on a young body, not to mention the caloric nightmare of dorm food....

I will be teaching you a few lifestyle tips. This book was written to help you live your natural college life and stay out of trouble, while maintaining your healthy well-being and your beautiful body. Have fun, learn, and be safe!

-Tim

FOREWORD

The transition from home life in high school to college is likely to be one of the most challenging milestones to face in one's life journey from youth towards personal independence.

The landscape is a new physical, emotional, and interpersonal surrounding. This handbook offers a stable foundation for the freshman entering college. Tim's perspective provides solid advice, sensible values and a simple framework for the social & emotional forces facing one's journey through the transition from adolescence to young adulthood.

Mr. Marsala's workout technique is sound from a structural, biomechanical and musculoskeletal viewpoint. His use of core body techniques coupled with offering three levels of difficulty (beginning, intermediate, and advanced) aid in achieving optimal fitness goals. His dietary recommendations are extremely enlightening, and the beverage advice will certainly make the college experience safe and rewarding.

-Armen S. Kelikian M.D.

Northwestern University Medical School, Professor of Orthopedic Surgery, Chicago, Il…. Consultant & Orthopedic Surgeon to the Chicago Bears

Acknowledgements

I would first like to thank my parents who have always supported my athletic endeavors as far back as I can remember, particularly in the realm of weightlifting. Leading up to my bodybuilding shows, my mother would always make sure the "proper" foods were prepared for me. My father was always great at landing workout equipment for our garage gym, not to mention their collective support and encouragement for me to compete. I couldn't have asked for two better role models.

After graduating from Eastern Illinois University in '97, I stumbled upon a job in the want adds of the Chicago Tribune. The Midtown Athletic Club was looking for qualified personal trainers to expand their staff. My only problem was that I was an unqualified personal trainer. I wasn't sure what to expect when it came time for an interview. So there I was sitting nervously in the club café and in walks the fitness manager, who little did I know, would have a profound influence on my career and life from that moment on.

His name is Duane Johnson and he is currently the club manager at Midtown. When Duane and I met, I don't think he looked at me and decided to be my mentor, it just kind of happened. Being new to the scene of personal training, I wasn't even sure what it meant to be a qualified or experienced instructor. After all, I was fresh out of college and knew everything (yeah right)! But there was something about Duane that I could identify with. There was something about him that challenged me to be the absolute best personal trainer that I could be. Maybe it was his verbal encouragement; maybe it was his ability to lead by example or his vast knowledge of 80s rock. Nonetheless, we developed a perfect student-teacher relationship that has helped get me where I am today. Thanks Duane!

Contributing Editors: Robin Campbell-Ouchida
                                          Paula Manta

Hair Stylist: Melisa Burdi of Zazu Salons
Graphic contributors: Tom Brunzelle and Adam Oliver
Photography: Dan Rowley
Illustrations: Natalie Mihok
Logo: Judith Barath www.judithbarathart.
                         com

TABLE OF CONTENTS

CHAPTER 1

CONGRATULATIONS ON YOUR COLLEGE ACCEPTANCE!

The chapter discusses: 1. Changes students frequently encounter upon transitioning into the college years: Leaving home and abandoning "comfort zones" (internal, social, emotional, and academic) 2. How to recognize and cope with commonly related issues such as homesickness, stress/anxiety, insomnia, and depression 3. Explaining the social polarities between Americans and that of other cultures (Why does their academic performance seem to be higher?) 4. Recommending a "New Balanced" attitude to pack in your bags necessary for embracing the stages of higher learning!

> *"The will to win, the desire to succeed, the urge to reach your full potential... these are the keys that will unlock the door to personal excellence."*

Ah... senior farewell...... The endless summer parties of exchanging stories and comparing the future paths of each "cage-freed" graduate.

"Yeah freedom... No more curfews! We can pick our classes and party whenever! .... Look: Underwater basket weaving 101..... Definitely on the list for the first semester! Told you guys *I* picked the right school," says your buddy laughing and displaying his fall course catalogue!

1

Then another classmate chimes in, pointing to her class schedule, "You're crazy, I'm taking twenty credits per semester! That way I'll definitely graduate in less than four years and get into med school early. See, this fall I'm signed up for two literature sections, calculus, physics, chemistry, and the multiple three hour labs included. How hard can this be?"

Okay, this may be how some high school grads perceive their collegiate futures, and yes, going away to school can appear quite idealistic, party-like, and glamorous for some. Perhaps the first fellow celebrating his departure may want to put a bit of curriculum into "his basket." Meanwhile the young lady with a schedule that exceeds the expectations of a medical student may need to realize that carrying a class load this heavy is unhealthy. She'll wind up studying in the cardiology unit all right…as a patient!

Contrarily, there are those realists who head back home from the post high school bash alone, developing a bit softer view. In reality, most grads are actually feeling a bit edgy about moving away from home and *still* haven't found an answer to the infinite question, "What do you want to be when you grow up?" It's O.K! …This is why universities offer undeclared majors.

There are a lot of pressures associated with leaving home. For starters, having to deal with bragging parents who have high expectations. "Oh my daughter is going to a 'Big 10' university, but she really had the scholarship over at the private liberal arts school in state… You know kids, they want to choose a college for fun times too, ha ha ha," you overhear your mother chuckling with the neighbors. "Great mom, thanks for the added pressure! What if I flunk out after three weeks," the daughter hollers back, storming off to her room.

Cheer up and go back to the party!

Hey you guys, remember Dr. Seuss's <u>Oh, The Places You'll Go!</u>?....
Well if you don't recall being recited any verses, pick it back up before
arriving at your new destination. Sure it may seem juvenile, but
hang-ups (or hangovers) and bang-ups (or bad bangs) can happen
to you!

Dr. Seuss continues to share that some days you'll feel on top of the
world, and other times you certainly will not. The important lesson
here is to learn and grow from life experiences, may they be positive
or devastating. I also agree with Charles Swindoll who says, "Life is
10% what happens to me and 90% how I react to it. And so it is with
you... we are in charge of our attitudes."

Now, let's get you: FIT, DRUNK? AND SMARTER!!!!

LEAVING YOUR COMFORT ZONE

Most of you are used to having a parent or guardian there (annoying
or not) providing meals, aiding with homework, doing your laundry,
or bailing you out of your latest "antic." Perhaps some of you have
significant mentors outside the home that you are used to relying
upon: special friends, siblings, teachers, or coaches. Or how about
leaving that high school sweetheart you swore you'd be faithful to
forever! Oops, too mushy...

I've had the recent pleasure of interviewing a football coach at one of
the local high schools here in the "burbs," both about his experience
being a student mentor, and his honest opinions about coaching:
Steve has been employed with the school district for over fifteen years
and frankly appeared burned out. He felt that his mental fatigue
wasn't because of the endless practices or traveling to away games,
but more so because of the students themselves. Fortunately I caught
him at the end of the day away from kids and his daily routine so he
could "vent" freely.

He said, "My brain is a host of many secrets accumulated over the years, all from students (both the boys and girls) who just don't feel comfortable confiding in parents or school social workers. I could write volumes of teen novels!" He continued to reveal their endless dramas, "The tears from unplanned pregnancies to abusive situations at home, to the fights amongst peers, to unfavorable report cards, and heart wrenching breakups. At this point, there is nothing I haven't heard from these kids! Sometimes I wonder why I didn't just become a social worker! When they finally do graduate and continue on to college, I write endless recommendations to ensure their future successes, but most importantly I let them know that Coach Steve is just a phone call away."

HOMESICKNESS

Remember leaving for summer camp that lasted one to two weeks at best? At first it was a blast with the campfires and canoe adventures! Yes, and by the end of week two, most of us were edgy to unpitch the tent and get back into our warm beds *at home!* ....UHHH College is a semester (or quarter) long and there's no jumping out of that tent (now the dorm)-just plunging into challenging classes, parties with strangers, and infinite hours in the library studying. For most, returning to our warm beds at home won't happen until the holidays, so homesickness is most likely going to occur at some time during the term. Don't feel ashamed. These reactions are completely natural and fortunately there are plenty of counselors on campus ready and anticipating your condition.

If you are unable to bond right away with the people at your new school, contact the Coach Steve type people back at home. Remember, leaving your comfort zone may be extremely difficult to tackle. Take their phone numbers and addresses with you to school. You never know when you'll need that old pep talk again.

EXPERIENCING STRESS AND ANXIETY

These are topics that will resurface over and over throughout the book! We know in today's world that <u>excessive amounts of stress</u> lowers our immune system, boosts the risk of heart disease, and generally contributes to us feeling unhealthy. Almost 90% of visits to primary care physicians today are due to stress-related problems. Because of this epidemic, the chapters will reveal multiple avenues for stress reduction (i.e. mainly through proper diet, alcohol and drug control/detoxification remedies, specific exercises, time management, and safe dating).

One way to realize you are stressed out or have anxiety is through symptoms such as: lack of sleep, a racing heartbeat, or maybe even by feeling sweaty. Initially, the short-term way to reduce stress is deep breathing, (a.k.a. diaphragmatic breathing). The second way to keep calm is to be realistic about your class load. Of course you're going to lose it if you're taking six courses your first semester. Don't emulate the girl quoted at the beginning of the chapter! College courses are a bit more challenging than high school classes, really.

Another way to keep calm is to GET TO CAMPUS EARLY! Yes, arrive at your dorm right when it opens (usually a few days or even a week before classes start). That way you can meet your R.A.s (residential advisors) who are ready for the typical edgy freshman behavior. Most schools have very beneficial programs pre-orientating and acclimating new students to college life. Also, try to become affiliated with groups on campus (i.e. Greek organizations, clubs within your major or intramural sports activities) Above all, avoid isolation and make time in your life for things that will calm you down!

GETTING TOO LITTLE SLEEP

Going to college can certainly promote sleep deprivation whether it's due to staying out partying all night, or finishing papers and studying for exams. Perhaps you're just stressed out from your new life away from home and can't seem to catch the zzzzzzz's. Maybe you have a roommate who snores or somehow prevents you from sleeping well no matter what you do. Whatever the reason, it can't continue. Being sleep deprived used to be considered a badge of honor where you'd hear, "Oh I stayed up all night cramming for that test," or, "It took me until 5:00 a.m. to finish that paper." Wrong! That translates into unhealthy procrastination.

In actuality, lack of sleep has been linked to such conditions as obesity, diabetes, high blood pressure and memory problems, even in young adults (i.e. YOU). So do what is necessary to get enough sleep each night. Otherwise it will interfere with the success of your college experience and long-term sleep deprivation can lead to illness. Get to the school infirmary if your sleeplessness continues. Remember each of us need at least 7-8 hours of sleep per night in order to function properly.

SOME TIPS FOR SLEEP AIDS:

1. Keep your bedroom clean and clutter-free (also keeps your mind free of excessive worry).
2. No Coffee or other caffeinated beverages late in the day
3. Avoid procrastinating schoolwork! It will cause you to stress out and stay up late trying to finish it.
4. Make sure your dorm room/sleeping space has the proper shades or blinds (dark enough). You are not a rooster!
5. Do not put a TV or other loud appliances next to where you are sleeping (remember, your mind is already distracted enough).
6. Try aromatherapy: Lavender and Chamomile teas are great options, but those ingredients are also in over-the-counter oils, lotions, and bath gels.
7. Lose the buzzer! Very important: set the alarm to awaken to soft music, not the annoying traditional shake you out of bed mode. The beeping, ringing and buzzing sounds have been proven to ignite internal stressors. The "noise" literally jolts the brain from a restful state into a cortisol releasing strain. Cortisol is the damaging hormone the body releases during trauma. This adrenal response is ideal when fleeing from a predator, but long-term release is harmful to the system. College can be stressful enough and being pulled out of a peaceful sleep is psychologically intrusive. Don't invite these unnecessary noises into your bed. Soft music will ease you out of REM...
8. If your roommate is a chronic snorer, discuss it with him/her. Perhaps you could agree to wear earplugs as long as he/she wakes you up in the morning.

Depression This condition continues to plague millions in our nation. It generally starts with feelings of being extremely overwhelmed or stressed out by some life experience. An individual with depression feels sad and of course, feeling sad is a natural emotion and part of human existence.

The difference between sad feelings and varying degrees of clinical depression is, sad feelings go away within a reasonable amount of time in a non-depressed person, whereas the sadness remains stagnant within depression. Many students with attention problems and learning disorders are especially susceptible to this condition, so if you are starting to feel lost in your classes GET HELP! Every college campus has a student health center that can help you get back on track.

Common side effects of depression include: sleep deprivation, weight gain or loss, headaches, or irritability. Some people may develop a lack of interest or prefer to withdraw from social everyday life situations. Understanding the difference between anxiety and depression is also very important, especially when you're young and away from family. Anxiety is when the individual is <u>too</u> revved up, whereas depression is experienced in the person who needs to become <u>more</u> energized or active. Both are treatable, but with different medications.

*** (Never borrow anyone else's prescribed medications for these conditions or any other! Each person reacts very differently to every medication). We will continue this topic in the next chapter relating specifically to drugs and alcohol.

CHAPERONE-FREE DATING

This topic certainly varies from student to student. Some are experienced with members of the opposite sex and then there are those students who are not. The point is, now that you've entered college, you are allowed to stay out with a date as late as you want and even sleep over at their pad if you choose to do so. There are no parents interviewing your dates, or popping into the family room making sure you're not smooching on the couch. Parents are not there to lecture you on when to be home and how sex is unacceptable under their roof! Some universities have gender and time restrictions, but most allow free will!

We will discuss safe dating and rape prevention to a greater extent in the both the guy's and girl's chapters educating students on how to experience positive dating situations throughout college.

New Curriculum

"What's a syllabus? Why isn't the bell ringing for class to start? Why are there two hundred people in this lecture hall? The last time I saw a room this big, I received my diploma in it! What if I have a question? There is no way in hell I'm going to raise my hand in a room full of this many students. Should I take notes? This is totally not what I expected. I'm used to eraser fights and passing notes. Hey, at least we can chew gum!"

After reading the syllabus and receiving the professor's preliminary ground rules, many think, "This is crazy! There is no way I can pass this class. How am I going to read six chapters a week in this boring book and actually remember it? Wow, I had a difficult time passing the chemistry final junior year, let alone getting through four years of classes like this." WELCOME TO COLLEGE!!...

Remember this exciting fact: "The more education you receive, the higher the earning potential in the future!" Interesting how certain cultures base their adolescent popularity on this quote.....

Who's popular in the other countries?

Many other societies (including people from India and those of Asian decent) place a strong emphasis upon academic success, while down playing the importance of landing a date with the hottest rack in class! Yes, everyone loves a pretty face or a chiseled figure (*all* are subject to human nature), but parents from these cultures instill a stronger sense of "delayed gratification" making playtime or social interaction secondary to learning and earning high GPA's.

According to <u>Top Of The Class</u> a new book revealing Asian and Asian American secrets of high academic achievement, their cultures now represent 20% of the Ivy League schools and 42% of Cal Berkley's student body, while only making up 4% of the U.S. population... Wow, they are definitely doing something right!

The authors share how a unique discipline exists, where children are *expected*, not asked, to do well in school. They understand that academic success is obligatory and crucial for the survival of their families! Praise is reserved for high achievement, not for a C-mediocre effort. Elders will not hesitate to point out the mistakes preventing youngsters from being *ahead* of the curve.

They are renowned for being tribal, where multiple generations collectively live under the same roof. The purpose is to keep their bloodlines infinite! They take care of grandparents/great-grandparents, have higher quantities of offspring, and educate their young to become strong providers.

This sense of high morality is carried over into the classroom and is shared amongst their peers, making it cool to do well in school. They do not find it amusing when a classmate is goofing off or failing a class, and disrespecting an instructor would be considered taboo.

CARRIED TOO FAR?

Unfortunately, some of these cultures have miserable gender inequalities. A higher value is placed upon male children, and in many nations women are still deprived of education. Observing the media related stories of female infant homicide and women having to cover their faces in public...is just infuriating! This is where *they* receive poor grades.

STEREOTYPICAL AMERICAN POPULARITY

Americans certainly prioritize literacy and fundamental education, but overachievers seem to represent a smaller percentage of our population. We place more emphasis on recreational activities and social interaction than the cultures mentioned above. Yes our country is the land of freedom and opportunity, but are we being *too* carefree? A Harvard acceptance letter is like practically wining the lottery, "Oh my God, What a total brain... What does he *look* like again?"

Most students in the U.S. put forth some degree of effort, but only to a limit. Not to insinuate laziness, but this mentality causes us to surrender our true capabilities. "I'm just not good at math. Oh well, at least my grades in English are okay." God forbid us to miss a smutty TV show, shopping, or the Friday night dance.

Lengthy visits with extended family (in-laws/grandparents) are considered *so* annoying, let alone cohabitating with them. "Hello, no way... company starts to stink after four days!" Not to say that we're selfish, but in the U.S. we value our "me time" and compromising such would be considered a loss.

Who do we deem popular in high school? Here's the Report Card:

A+ ....Looks (Face & Body)
A.............Cool and expensive clothes, hairstyle, cell phone,
A.............Achievement in sports, class office, cheerleading, or earning the crown!
B+ .... $$ and a cool car
B .... Being witty/funny or life of the party
B- .... The total brain that helped *me* with a paper

THE SUCCESSFUL "NEW BALANCE"

Not only is this the brand of tennis shoe I wear and recommend to clients, it dictates the operation of my everyday Libra existence. Balance and moderation are the keys to a healthy lifestyle. Too much of *anything* isn't good. Excessive food consumption will make you ill, while obsessive running can rupture a knee. The same holds true with the cultural differences discussed. Academic success coupled with strong family values are a must, but the gender inequalities need to be flushed. *Everyone* should be given the same chances and opportunities in life. Simultaneously, the superficial shopping and dances need to be tossed on the back burner!

Your new profs are not going to set the curve based upon who has the grandest tiara or biggest muscles. Frankly, the way instructors reward high grades is through participation and effort. By the way, they *do* know whether you are showing up to class or not! Obviously if a person enjoys a topic enough to eventually teach it, they are remotely interested in whom the audience is. You don't have to become an overnight protégé, however, you should at least try expressing an interest in *their* class….. And… just from observation, instructors really loathe the dingy "I didn't know" routine.

In order to be successful we *have to* prioritize school over our social lives!

Think of it this way, we would all love to devour ice cream sundaes for three square meals and toss fiber to the cattle! Great… we'd all buzz around overweight and diabetic with uncontrollable road rage. Wait a minute. That *is* our society, oops! (Of course maintaining proper health will be addressed in the dietary section listing strategies to avoid those conditions). The point being, we first have to ingest the proper nutrients for our bodies to function properly. Then as a reward (once in a while), have the dessert.

Our life choices require the same prioritization. If you are constantly gabbing on your cell phone instead of studying for mid-terms, your grades will become "unhealthy" rendering you to failure. Get your studying and papers out of the way, and then socialize.

Please remember that *all* people are equal in the eyes of God. If you want to be a professional waitress, guess what? You won't have to study very much. Now if your dream is to become a physician….. *All* med students spend the majority of their lives with their heads buried in textbooks! I once asked a brilliant physician how much time he had spent in school. Rolling his eyes he replied, "Forever. I put my blood sweat and tears into this practice!" Titles and degrees aren't just handed to us; we have to earn them, people! You control your future….. "Life is 1% inspiration & 99% perspiration!" –Thomas Jefferson

In <u>The Seven Spiritual Laws of Success</u> Deepak Chopra (renowned eastern *and* western spiritual guru) contributes to our successful New Balance by offering the following advice: The three components to the Law of Dharma "purpose in life:"

1. Each of us is here to discover our true *higher* Self…..

2. *Every* human being has a unique talent that no one else possesses…

3. We all need to serve humanity. Don't think "What's in it for me?" Instead ask yourself, "How can I help? Or… How can I help those that I come into contact with?"

CHAPTER 2

GETTING YOUR DRINK ON!

Understanding alcohol (and other party enhancing substances)

The chapter will inform the reader of: 1. The physiological effects of alcohol, drugs, and cigarettes upon the body 2. The body's natural inflammatory response to substances (hangovers and our immune system) 3. Legal truths of alcohol and drugs (includes valuable advice from defense attorney Donald Ramsell) 4. The nutritional reality of your cocktails (The caloric values and proofs of hard alcohol, beer, wine, mixers, etc. 5. Which drinks and mixers put the weight on and elevate B.A.C. (Blood Alcohol Content) 6. Safety <u>musts</u> while consuming alcohol/ "partying."

"Don't ya hate Perry's wife"- Arthur 1982

Drinking in college is just going to happen! Outside of routine library visits and exams, alcohol consumption seems to creep its way into almost all events: hall parties, sports tailgaters, post-midterm celebrations, 50 cent beer nights at the local saloon....and the list goes on. Where did this ritualistic behavior come from? If the classes are now *more* difficult than high school, why are we killing *more* brain cells? Seems a bit perverse doesn't it? Perhaps it's just students exercising the freedom factor, "See mom and dad, look what I can do now.... hic-up!" Or... maybe it's just good old fashioned peer pressure mixed with a bit of inter-campus tradition. Who knows?

Anyway, what we do know for sure is that most college kids *do* party and we're not here to psychoanalyze anyone, just trying to instill a safe and healthier lifestyle.

Of course flicks like "Animal House" are the extreme example with Belushi in his toga, pounding booze, and smashing his fraternity bro's guitar against the wall. The movie paints a one dimensional, wild picture of college life: drinking and portraying failure as funny. Although in Belushi's defense the guy *did* sing I Gave My Love a Cherry. Anyone would throw a fit after that painful ballad.

It's certainly O.K. to have a screwball personality, but don't let the partying sink your brain into a 0.0 GPA, and please at least remember that the Germans did *not* bomb Pearl Harbor! Great movie, but don't make it your reality.

Now there are those students who choose not to drink. Wow, hats off to you! Both your parents and your liver thank you. Feel free to read along with the drunks, perhaps you will gain some knowledge as to why your puking dorm mates are packing on the "freshman 15" faster than you. Obviously you will benefit more from the workout and dietary chapters, but please review some of the mixers for they may pertain to your "virgin drinking" lifestyle.

The Physiological Effects of Alcohol
Now as for you connoisseurs of the mind-altering world, there is an obligation to your parents, the universities, and obviously you to provide a brief lecture on the negative effects and ramifications of drinking alcohol. Many apologies to those bio-chemistry majors for this may appear quite remedial for your talented scientific minds........

"No" to alcohol
According to Webster's New Collegiate Dictionary, alcohol is: "A colorless volatile flammable liquid C_2H_5OH that is the intoxicating agent in fermented and distilled liquors- called also ethyl alcohol..."

Wow that's harsh. Volatile? Flammable? Didn't you expect a softer definition? Maybe something like, "A substance consumed for centuries utilized to promote relaxation and lower social inhibitions... sometimes it comes from a potato and is available in a variety of colors and fruit flavors.... sort of like fluoride."

Alright.... a bit goofy, but it's just so hard to envision a cold brewski on Friday night being volatile, let alone flammable. So after the Webster's wake up call, I was inspired to dig into further research regarding our favorite spirits, and unfortunately found multiple studies unveiling booze as being extremely toxic to the body.

According to <u>Life Extension Disease Prevention and Treatment</u>, it's best to never expose the body to alcohol in any quantity. Alcohol in surplus depletes essential anti-oxidants (disease fighters), while sending a flood of *free radicals attacking the brain, immune system, vital organs, and skin layers. They even go as far as comparing excessive alcohol intake to that of radiation poisoning, and consequently if one does choose to consume, it's certainly recommended to do so in moderation. (1)

*free radicals
This medical encyclopedia revealed inflammation and free radical damage as culprits for the negative effects of alcoholic beverages. Free radicals are the cell-destroying, unstable molecules lacking an electron created both from inflammatory response, and its own sources and within our environment (cigarette smoke, air pollution, sunlight, and through alcohol consumption). They are literally magnetized or drawn to other stable molecules because they possess the electrons free radicals are deprived of.(2)

The Inflammation Process...
Is the response of tissues within the body caused by irritation or injury (displayed physically through pain, swelling, redness, and heat). It's generally brought on by viral or bacterial infections, although inflammatory response can also arise through the over-consumption of toxins and chemicals ingested or absorbed, which

have accumulated over time. The body responds through an implosive reaction by means of the impairment and destruction of multiple cells. (3)

Consuming alcohol in high quantities will send the same alarming inflammatory message directly to the cells throughout the body. Your system registers excessive booze intake as toxic, needing to eliminate it A.S.A.P. This is the reason why a "hangover" exists: The body reacts exactly as if it were being poisoned, hence the medical term "alcohol poisoning." The cells become swollen and heated (inflamed) from drinking heavily, leading to their individual destruction. Any time the body is in this "state," it's considered to be catabolic, or deteriorating (4)

Here's an example….. What happens when you get a splinter in your finger?

Well, primarily it hurts. Secondly, your finger becomes heated, turns red, and sometimes starts to bleed. This is your body's response to the intrusion. It simply does not want a foreign piece of wood lodged under its skin. Your system will do everything within its biological power to kick this invading object out, i.e. sending blood directly to the area, creating a flushing effect revealed as redness and swelling. This is why long-term drinkers have red noses or faces. Alcohol is like a digested splinter spread throughout the body.

Dehydration
Another *lovely* consequence of consuming alcohol! Maintaining hydration, for all living organisms, is essential for survival. The human body is composed of over 70% water, and just like plants and flowers, if we do not water ourselves we too will die. Drinking literally shuts off the hormone responsible for retaining fluids in the body. This is why we frequently urinate after hitting the keg. This alone will cause the body to require a significant amount of replenishment, let alone if you wind up praying to the porcelain God (puking). See the detoxification chapter for proper hydration tips.

The Thymus Gland
Located in the lower portion of the neck, the Thymus is considered the master gland. Its chief responsibility is to manufacture and maintain T-Cells and white blood cells. These cells are vital for fighting off both bacterial and viral infections. If the gland malfunctions in any way, the immune system becomes inhibited and the production of T-Cells and white blood cells is halted. Excessive alcohol consumption will literally cause this gland to shrink, rendering us vulnerable to disease and premature aging (5).

The Liver
The liver stores and regulates blood throughout the entire body. It is also in control of flexing and extending the joints and muscles. The nature of this organ is to grow and disperse. Both its expansion and function are literally inhibited by alcohol consumption. Not only does booze directly eat away at the organ, but it prevents the liver from doing its job of eliminating toxins from the body (6).

Hormonal Imbalances
Drinking alcohol in excess will also obstruct the liver's enzymatic activity, necessary for hormonal regulation. It causes testosterone to be converted into estrogen, which can be extremely contaminating in the body (7).

Glutathione Depletion
Alcohol inhibits the production of this essential protein produced in the liver. Glutathione is the chief antioxidant that not only protects individual cells, but aids to strengthen the tissues of the arteries, brain, heart, immune cells, liver, kidneys, lungs and skin. It fights cancer and the most detrimental free radical damage (8).

Vitamin and Mineral Depletion
These essentials become hindered, rendering us more vulnerable to disease and infection (i.e. Vitamin B1 thiamine is essential for neutralizing alcohol by-products and protecting against cellular damage, becomes depleted through excessive alcohol consumption).

Worsens Depression

For some students, college can bring about symptoms of depression due to homesickness or feeling overwhelmed by a challenging new curriculum. If you are experiencing some form of depression or anxiety, drinking to excess may worsen the condition. Remember, alcohol is classified as a depressant drug. (9)

Cheers

Now that everyone is afraid to drink, let's view our second opinion....

On the other side of the global consensus, many agree that one to two drinks per day (preferably red wine) may have positive effects upon the body. Foster's <u>Detox Solutions</u> reveals moderate drinking to be beneficial promoting positive circulation and cardiovascular function. Alcohol may also serve as a cellular anti-oxidant (the grape seed extract in wine), and thorough studies have revealed that people who consume one to two drinks per day actually endured *less* illness and lived longer than those who avoided alcohol completely.(10)

*Never applaud smoking

Sorry chimneys, there are zero studies supporting your filthy habit. Free radicals and toxins are hosted in the everyday air we breathe and are multiplied when cigarette smoke is present (mainly through the combination of oxygen with carbon monoxide). It's amazing just how detrimental and aging this habit can be. (11)

More than one-fifth of U.S. adults, or 46 million people, are actively smoking, according to the Centers for Disease Control and Prevention. If you haven't taken up this nasty habit, then don't! To reduce your susceptibility for illness, risks of cancer and early aging try switching over to the patch or over-the-counter nicotine gum. In a review of 123 studies published in 2004, nicotine gum and other replacement treatments such as the patch upped the odds of being able to quit two times compared to relying on willpower alone.

Remember in science class where we learned about the exchange of oxygen (O_2) and carbon dioxide (CO_2) between plants and people? If we're inhaling cigarette smoke (CO) when we're supposed to be inhaling the O_2 from plants necessary for survival, when does the body rid itself of toxins and CO_2? How does the system rid itself of pollutants? It doesn't!

Can't we always point out the chain smoker in the room? Obviously the smell gives them away, but how does their face look? Usually it's discolored, dry, red, blotchy, with dark circles under the eyes revealing obvious signs of poor circulation. This literally comes from A LACK OF OXYGEN (O_2).

Not only does this habit lead to a dependency on nicotine, but it accelerates avenues of internal inflammation leading to poor health, and yes, smoking does cause cancer! Inhaling secondhand smoke is just as bad. Couple secondhand cigarette smoke with everyday environmental pollutants.... it presents the same contaminating free-radical damage as if you were the smoker.

Puffing away doesn't reflect the cool James Dean or Sharon Stone image anymore. All it creates is an unpleasant stench in your mouth, hair, and clothing! Plus, it compounds a hangover by contributing more toxins to your bloodstream.

*Chewing/dipping isn't any better... similar contaminants enter the body!

To avoid tobacco contamination:

1. Buy the patch or gum
2. Work out (see chapter on exercise)
3. Limit time in smoke-filled places
4. See dietary chapter (internal cleansing)

> *"Killer Bees!"*
> -Chris Farley in "Tommy Boy"

Legal Ramifications

Drinking and Driving

Ouch, another terrible habit! Drinking impairs your ability to drive more than you know. Vehicular collisions and homicide are almost always alcohol-related. Please don't drink and drive. Decades of statistics have proven that someone *will* get injured or killed. It's expected that designated driver situations will fall through from time to time, but don't play tough guy/gal! "Oh I'm fine. I only drank beer and besides I drive better after a couple." Yadda Yadda… The death scare tactic works with most, but there are still some immortals out there who feel the effects of drinking and driving don't apply to them. Hmmmm, maybe this will work:

Bet I can get you to stop drinking and driving... Ready?

Have you ever noticed that cops have laptop computers mounted in between the "shotgun" and the steering wheel? Uhhh …what do you suppose they're doing? … Emailing a friend? ... Perhaps creating a sequel to this book? …Or maybe writing a letter of appreciation to the local donut shop? Yeah right… dream and read on!

Hate to blow any "under cover" covers, but they are running any and all license plate numbers through in their laptop friends! Yes, and while the squad car is still following close behind, they're able to miraculously retrieve the registered owner's personal driving record. This is a great strategy if there happens to be an estranged murderer on the loose, but not for trapping everyday civilians.

"What, they can't do that! That's total entrapment," you reply! Oh yes they can. Your "big brother" from another mother is a COP! "He" can perform this investigation whenever "he" deems necessary. So, what if you are driving a vehicle whose owner was convicted of prior D.U.I. charges? What if the owner's license is or was suspended? Guess who they're pulling over? Better hope you haven't been drinking.

Don't take it personally; this is just standard police procedure today. What if you really did forget to signal right? What if your car had a tail light out? By the way, what time are you leaving the bar or party, probably pretty late right? After 10:00 P.M. cops *expect* that drivers have been drinking. Besides, do you think maybe the police are waiting outside of bars for people to stumble into their cars? Shark-infested waters, kids! They don't care if it's your first time, or you were just driving your *drunker* roommate home. Your busted ass increases their chance of promotion!

It gets worse?
Here's another eye opener: Did you know we are going towards a national driver's license, no longer state mandated? This makes any previous record *impossible* to hide. Plus D.U.I. charges do *not* drop off your record anymore. They used to be like speeding tickets, dissolving after a few years. Now court systems dig back twenty plus years if need be to find a prior...Yes, be scared! They want *your* revenue and the laws are becoming harsher each year. So...

1. Wake up and walk home with a buddy, *not alone* (you probably need to burn the extra booze calories anyway)

   Or....

2. Call a cab (much cheaper than a $5,000.00 D.U.I. charge)

See.... Knew I could stop ya from boozing and cruising! .....Harsh reality, but remember this book is here to make you smarter in *all* aspects of college life.

I just got caught... What can I do about it now?

Sorry if this F.Y.I. is a bit late. Hopefully you don't learn *everything* the hard way. At least you know how to avoid arrests in the future.

But at this point the only way to lighten or dismiss any charges is to GET A LAWYER!! On many occasions an attorney will find loopholes in a case where the officer has forgotten to follow everyday protocol (i.e. failing to conduct sobriety tests correctly or not reading specific documents). The charges may get thrown out.

At the same time, a judge will hold your case in much higher regard if you're in court with a legal professional. Please do not try to fight your own case, even if you are in law school. "Flying solo" is perceived as disrespectful and frankly annoying to a judge. It's like attending a country club without a member where you're destined to crash! Court prosecutors, judges, district attorneys, and defense counsel all operate intricately in a fraternal fashion to handle cases like yours. Following *their* club rules is a crucial part of this <u>not</u> so fun process. Take an experienced and "invited" member with you!

*According to Illinois Top D.U.I. Attorney Donald Ramsell, "A person who attends court without legal representation might as well walk up to the Judge's bench and ask to have their head chopped off!" Quite the visual…. and unfortunately it's true. The charges D.U.I. offenders receive today are brutal: The loss of a driver's license, jail time, and hefty fines….UGGG! So, you might as well try to fight it (with a lawyer), the charges can't get any worse. Besides you're *already* going to be handed a nasty bill for the damages. (12)

On a positive note, you will certainly gain insight into our legal system, especially if your case does go to trial. Try not to personalize any of this and <u>don't</u> become a cop hater. The boyz in blue are here for our protection as well… However, there is a degree of entertainment that comes along with watching a mentally challenged officer being cross examined by a slippery defense. …It may just "turn that frown upside down!"

Above all, don't stress… This too shall pass!!

*Through the national website <u>www.dialdui.com</u>, Ramsell offers valuable information including: Case highlights, Court penalties, and **40 ways to beat a DUI…**

Sorry guys, brutal section. Tell me about it… this is the WORST! You do have to admit though this stuff *is* pretty darn enlightening. Whomever believes ignorance is bliss has either never been pulled over or just lives in a bubble. You didn't really think this book was about sit-ups and avoiding jelly doughnuts… did you?

O.K. Catch your breath yet? Come on, back in the legal ring. Let's recall counselor Ramsell back to the stand…

21 Yet?
No, well then the sirens are still apt to turn on. Again? Yep. Guess who else knows you're underage? That would be the protective staff dressed in blue peering through the windows into your Friday night celebration and they would *love* to eyeball an identifiable beer can "you're just holding for your 21 year old friend." The proper title for this misdemeanor charge is Minor In Possession (MIP)…. This notorious ticket is incredibly expensive and is accompanied by the loss of your driver's license until you really are 21. And since you are in the 18 and over group, this fresh misdemeanor charge will be a permanent brand on your record! (13)

Minor or Adult?
The last time we checked, the vast percentage of college students are between the ages of 18 and 20. In terms of unfair double standards and legal susceptibility, these three years are horrible. Not to promote drinking amongst this age group, but ya'll have it bad. We allow an 18-year-old "adult" to drive a car, go to war, and operate a semi automatic weapon… at their sexual peak! But when that same 18-year-old takes one sip of beer, that "adult" who is tried as an "adult" in a court of law, receives a "minor" in possession charge? I don't get it either! Anyway, my heart goes out to you!

By the way, if these cops are required to meet a quota in a tiny college town, don't you think they're apt to know where the big tickets are? Not to imply that anyone is a trust funder, but most cops assume your parents are paying for your mistakes, and the "legal tab." If you are one of those young "adults" who chooses to drink, don't stand anywhere near a window and definitely drink out of a sippy cup. After all you are a minor!

> *"Beetlejuice, Beetlejuice, Beetlejuice!"*
> *- Winona Rider " BeetleJuice"*

Fake ID's

Red Flag! Felony! You're better off with the D.U.I. Whether you've altered your own driver's license or just borrowing some 21-year-old's who resembles you, if a cop catches you... you are beyond busted! Not only will you have a felony charge on your permanent "adult" record, but just like the MIP, the courts will revoke your driving privileges until you do turn 21. (14)

Drugs

Oh wow, cops love pill poppers too! Yes let's revisit the spine crawling lecture. Still completely illegal, drugs and their possession charges are relentless. Most are felony related. You do not want a criminal record. It makes it nearly impossible to get a job. The securities industry will not hire you, and forget about law or medical school. If you are becoming addicted to drugs or alcohol, seek a physician's help.

Most non-prescribed drugs are hazardous to your health! Be careful they can be laced with or contain foreign contaminants (i.e. formaldehyde, rat poisoning etc....). Drugs like ecstasy "rolling" can cause severe impairment or fatality if mixed with alcohol.
Remember the synergistic effect from health class? When you combine drugs and/or alcohol, they are likely to have compounding effects. Not that I've ever inhaled marijuana, but when you mix a few puffs with the liquor you've already consumed.......it's lights out!

Many of the doctor-prescribed drugs such as antidepressants, anti-anxiety meds, and mood stabilizers become intensified or nullified (they either don't work as well or not at all) when combined with alcohol. Most of these prescriptions specify on the label: "Do not consume alcohol while taking this medication." This is not a suggestion, it's a warning! Please remember, don't ever take someone else's prescribed medication. It could have a completely different effect on you! (15)

Caloric Realities of Your Cocktails (**All alcohol calorie values are approximate)

Alcohol	Proof	Calories
Beer (12 oz.)		
Reg draft	9-10	130-160
Lite	8-9	100-115
Malt	12-13	160-175
Stouts/Ales	11-14	150-210
Wine (5 oz)		
Red (dry)	24-26	100-120
White (dry)	24-26	100-120
Sweeter wines	24-26	200-226
Liqueurs (1.5oz)		
Crème de Menthe	40	185
Peppermint Schnapps	40	125
Hard Alcohol (1.0 oz)		
Rum	100	125
	94	115
	80	85
Whisky	100	125
	94	115

Southern Comfort	80	144
Vodka	94	115
	100	125
Tequila	80	115

Diagram 1.1

MIXED DRINKS (1.0 OZ HARD ALCOHOL W/4OZ-6OZ OF MIX)

Bloody Mary: 115 calories
Gin & Tonic: 171 calories
Pina Colada: 262 calories
Whiskey Sour: 122 calories

You get the idea...

BEER

To this day I love Oktoberfest as much as the next guy or gal with all of those delicious seasonal brews! These beers, along with Guinness and Bass ales, are meant to be consumed in lower quantities, and treated like fine wines. They are rich in taste, hence being higher in calories and alcohol content.....not meant to beer bonged!

Tip: Squeeze and throw in a *lemon! Not only does this enhance the flavor, it adds nutrients to the beer (They are high in vitamin C) and low in calories. Lemons also have natural anti-septic properties, which helps ward off colds and influenza.

*Please do not confuse the lemons in beer with the toxic, booze-filled fruit in "jungle juice."

JUNGLE JUICE

The notorious punch hosting *scary* ingredients ... From recollection, I do believe this is a concoction incorporating sugar, every sweet fruit juice and cut up pieces of fruit all to offset the powerful taste of Ever Clear or Bacardi 151. Yes, this is probably one of the fastest ways to get loaded because it tastes so good and you can hardly detect any alcohol!

Now here's the "Webster's flammable." Yes those are the two types of alcohol that you can literally start a fire with! Remember the beginning of the movie "Revenge of the Nerds" where the AB brothers were performing fireballs? The fraternity house literally burned to the ground. Another hilarious movie, but please don't invite those flames into your living space. There's nothing worse than a drunken pyromaniac!

Don't eat the fruit!
You probably think you're being healthy by snacking on the fresh pieces of fruit floating in the punch bowl, right? Eating to absorb some of the alcohol you're consuming? How deceiving, the fruit probably has significantly higher alcohol content than the juice itself. Your host has most likely been marinating it in Ever Clear overnight. Sorry to blow the cover of those "gentlemen" trying to get girls overly intoxicated at parties. Remember we are trying to promote safety in this book.

Don't shoot the messenger on this, just delivering the facts. You decide whether you want to expose your vital organs to this party punch.

> 6 OZ. = Approximately 350 calories
> 60 grams of sugar
> Proof of Alcohol 151-200

*Mixer (8 oz.)	*Calories	Fat
Juice Apple Orange Grapefruit Cranberry	110-160	0 grams
Vegetable	50-60	0 grams
Regular Soda Cola 7-Up	100-130	0 grams
Margarita mix	110-120	0 grams
Tom Collins mix	110-120	0 grams
Egg Nog	Just buy the fat free kind during the holidays	

Diagram 1.2

*Try alternating these with some of the calorie-free flavored waters

*(B.A.C.) Blood Alcohol Content: Percentage of alcohol in the bloodstream

The legal driving limit for *all* states is below .08

Percentage	**Level of Impairment
.05	Lowered inhibitions The "who cares?" begins
.15	Cognitive reasoning is extremely inhibited
.25	Poor decision making Extreme slurring & Stumbling
.40	Passed out or in the E.R. (Death is possible)

Diagram 1.3

*According to the University of Oklahoma Police Department, the B.A.C. is determined through four factors: 1. Quantity of drinks consumed; 2. What you are drinking; 3. How much you weigh; 4. How many hours you've been drinking (16)
**The level of impairment is approximated

*Examples:

Quantity	*Type of Drink	Weight	# of hours drinking	B.A.C.
5 Drinks	12oz regular draft beer	200lbs/120lbs	2	.06/.09
5 Drinks	5oz glass of wine	200lbs/120lbs	2	.07/.12
5 Drinks	1oz 80 proof hard alcohol (shot/on the rocks/ mixed drink)	200lbs/120lbs	2	.07/.12
5 Drinks	Dry Martini	200lbs/120lbs	2	.14/.24

----

*All scenarios are approximated(17)

How to Consume Healthier and Safer

As a thirty-three year old college grad, I've had the opportunity of seeing both sides of the intoxifying spectrum. There have certainly been plenty o' evening of throwing back and practically winding up in a dumpster. At the same time I've witnessed plenty of scenes working as a bouncer in school. We've all been there sloshed leaving the local pub, but when you're the sober spectator, it isn't exactly the same funny picture. In fact, there really isn't anything amusing about watching a pretty girl with eye make-up smeared on her face, stumbling and slurring out the door. Or how about the sweet kid from down the hall developing beer muscles and picking fights over the pool table?

Tips for safe drinking:

1. Know and understand how to keep your B.A.C. (Blood Alcohol Content) within a safe range (see charts above)

2. Always eat a full meal before drinking

3. Drink one 8oz. glass of water for every alcoholic beverage consumed

4. Never leave your drink unattended! You never know who's scoping you out.

   (A good friend of mine went to the same university as Scott Peterson *and* another lived two blocks down from Jeffrey Dahmer during his feasting years!) The "Mickies" and "Date Rape" drugs slipped into cocktails are classified as animal tranquilizers!

5. Follow the classic safety in numbers buddy system. Always go out with trustworthy and reliable friends

6. Don't eat the fruit in Jungle Juice! You won't be able to gage your B.A.C.

CHAPTER 3

BEFORE THE AFTER PARTY

This chapter discusses: 1. Symptoms of the drinking aftermath! 2. Tips to repair the "hangover" damage: including a. The detoxification process b. The vitality of water and hydration c. Pain relievers d. Purifying food remedies & e. for exercise 3. Pre-partying strategies to avoid a nasty morning after...

"Oh... You can do it!" – Rob Schneider

"The Water Boy"

Top of da "mourning" to ya! ....
Not to imply that you're recovering from a St. Patrick's Day Bash, although a four-leafed clover would probably come in handy about now......especially if you overslept and missed your 8:00 class. Hopefully the drunken' stupor didn't cause you to miss an exam or important speech.... Don't forget our successful "New Balance" now: You're supposed to prioritize your collegiate career and leave the junk food (or drinking) as a *secondary* reward!

By the way, the "balancing-act" reminder will be resurfacing throughout the chapters! I *do* have a vested interest here. Eventually you cats will be running our nation and... frankly I'd feel a whole lot better knowing our future leaders had their priorities straight! ....Can you imagine a president who couldn't speak any "fantastical" English? or... How about one so busy with girlies that he could actually miss terrorists creeping into the country? Talk about toxins.... Let's *not* let this happen shall we?

Speaking of toxins… Are you ready to assess your painful *morning?*

Why do I feel so awful?
Remember the lecture on inflammation and free radical damage? Uhh well, that would be you right about now. Your body is reacting to the poisoning effects of alcohol consumption. Drinking to excess will cause the body to malfunction and produce the following notorious symptoms:

Headache?
Outside of literally causing brain damage, your high octane beverages have switched off that hormone vital for retaining water in the body… This dehydration coupled with enflamed brain cells will equate to a pounding migraine!

Nausea?
A bit gross, but as you know… the body only has a few ways to expel unwanted materials. Vomiting is certainly one of them. As a matter of fact this may still happen this morning, or maybe it already did last night? When we ingest alcohol, the first organ to react is the stomach. *It releases histamine known to irritate the stomach lining and cause pain and nausea. Don't worry there are remedies and this feeling won't last forever… unless of course you drink heavily again!

*Please try to avoid consuming alcohol if you have an ulcer or ulcer-like symptoms. Booze will worsen the condition.

Sweating?
Outside of urinating and vomiting, this is another way the body rids itself of pollutants, toxins, or bacteria. Don't we typically perspire during a period of illness or high fever? "Sweating out a hangover" is similar, except you've made yourself sick.

Shaky?
Hate to use the word "withdrawals" so early in your drinking career, but that jittery feeling is a combination of toxic overload and your neuro-chemistry being thrown off-balance. Alcohol consumption is effective for increasing GABA (Gamma-aminobutyric acid) the

amino acid found in the central nervous system (especially the brain). GABA possesses a natural sedative effect, essential for curbing chronic stress and anxiety. It inhibits neurotransmitter function by slowing nerve transmission.(1) This is why we find people saying, "I need a drink" after a long and stressful day or situation. Alcohol provides a *temporary* relief from life's perceived discomforts.

Many experts have noted that individuals who are more irritable or "high strung" tend to experience worse hangover symptoms. It makes sense… If a person is naturally deficient in GABA, robbing more of this calming amino acid from the body (the post drinking state) will compound stress and irritability.

Be Careful… alcohol is extremely addicting!
By drinking continuously, the brain does not have enough time to repair and return to its natural state. If you keep training the body to need booze in order to feel good, than eventually you will become conditioned to drink just to feel normal, let alone "happy." Don't worry I won't use the "A" word, only warning you against alcohol addiction. (2)

Dizzy?
No blonde joke intended, just referring to the other "light-headed" state. Maybe you're a bit sleep deprived, but most likely it's the depressant drug (alcohol) you've consumed to excess making you feel this way. Experts say that every time alcohol is consumed, thousands of brain cells are sacrificed… Feeling "Brain Dead?" It's because….You are!

You have none of the symptoms mentioned above? …. Maybe you're still drunk!

You don't remember?
This means you are having blackouts! Sorry, no time for sugar coating here… NOT GOOD! If this is becoming a repeated occurrence, something has to change… and fast. This is scary stuff here… *Anything* can happen to you! Not to bog you down with horrifying

statistics, but the number of date rapes is at an all time high, and STD's aren't something you want to be catching or passing around. Certain diseases (i.e. HIV/AIDS) are incurable at this point and are contracted by many people under the age of 25...

By the way, this "high risk" behavior will give you a bad reputation! Yes universities have far more students, but eventually lush-like or sleazy behavior will spread...and usually to the wrong people. What if you meet someone relationship worthy? ... The *last* thing you need are the grotesque echoes of last weekend being whispered in his/her ear! Clean up you act or you *will* pay for it.... one way or another. Please refer back to the B.A.C. chart and learn to gage your drinking. If you *still* can't eliminate blackouts, than quitting is probably the only option!

TAKING CARE OF YOURSELF AFTER THE PARTY

Detox is a Must!
Welcome to the world of detoxification. Don't worry, this does not mean we're sending you to rehab... Detoxing is the body's natural cleansing process especially important for eliminating the self-induced damage from the night before (or two+ nights) depending on how long you've been hitting the bottle! Remember the painful splinter used to illustrate inflammation? Detox works in conjunction with the inflammatory response to get rid of unwanted chemicals and toxins accumulated throughout the body. (3)

The exit path
Food and beverages are initially processed through the stomach and small intestines, but the liver and kidneys are responsible for the major processing and disposal of toxins. Once food is ingested, the intestines sort out the essential nutrients from toxins where the useful products are absorbed into the body, while harmful chemicals are sent to the detox system. (4)

Over 70% of these toxins are *non water-soluble* and sent directly to the liver, where they are neutralized with natural enzymes and made water-soluble. When the body is overloaded with toxins (i.e. excessive alcohol consumption) the liver becomes unable to filter and process them all. As a bodily safety mechanism, the excess toxins are stored into fat cells.(5)

As for the toxins that are neutralized and made water-soluble by the liver, they are transferred into the bowel and kidneys to continue the filtration process. This is a major reason we need to drink water... maintaining proper hydration enables the body to successfully complete the flushing process... and the final exit path? That would be your finding the closest toilet or bush. (6)

Please Don't start taking your detox organs for granted because unfortunately they become extremely taxed after each cocktail-filled event... to the point where they suffer in silence. If we could see through the abdominal wall and witness the damage alcohol inflicts upon our organs, prohibition would certainly be reinstated.

*Consuming foods that are high in anti-oxidants, high in fiber, and promote anti-inflammation will reverse a lot of the damage.

*See chapter 4 to view these foods

Start at the faucet!
No, not to fill up water balloons, although an absolutely phenomenal way to irritate your R.A.! You need to *drink* the water ... out of a cup.... and a lot of it! It's time to replenish the water that your keg-filled tailgaters (or other cocktails) have extracted from your body. Booze literally sucks you dry!

Here's an analogy (See... S.A.T's are useful): What happens to a refreshing cucumber after you've saturated it in salt, vinegar, and spice? It shrivels, shrinks, and eventually becomes a condiment. After an evening of countless drinks, a person becomes that "marinated" cucumber! Haven't you ever heard your parents say, "My, they certainly look *pickled?*" They were referring to someone's post-booze state.

So… marinade is to cucumber… as….. booze is to body

Every other magazine spills the evidence that we need to drink 8-10 8oz. glasses of water per day in order to maintain healthy bodily function. Water flushes toxins out of individual cells promoting optimal health and…. **weight loss** yeah!! Multiple studies also reveal that not only does drinking alcohol contribute to dehydration, but many other factors do as well including: extreme temperatures, lengthy exposure to the sun, caffeinated beverages, and foods high in sodium… All of which require us to increase our daily requirements. For every beverage containing alcohol or caffeine, we need to consume one 8 oz. glass of water.(7)

Oddly enough, people are still not fulfilling their daily water quotas. Maybe the "8-10 glasses" law is a bit too vague. Let's put it into perspective… Obviously a 30-pound child wouldn't need to drink ten glasses of water per day… or else their potty training would fall directly in the toilet. At the same time, a 260 lb. + individual actually needs to consume *more* than the recommended amount in order to remain hydrated and "flushed." To make it simple, just consume ½ your body weight in water per day. So if you weigh 120 lbs, drink at least *six* 8oz. glasses daily. If you weigh 300 lbs, you're drinking a minimum of *fifteen glasses*….Wow if that isn't an incentive to keep the weight off, I don't know what is?

By the way, lying around in a swimming pool does not count as part of your daily quota. You aren't a plant. Water doesn't just soak in through your feet! It needs to be ingested orally or delivered intravenously, and I'm *sure* you don't have access to hospital equipment (better not) so it's down the hatch. Besides the chlorine in your little "oasis" is dehydrating in and of itself… You're better off hanging with frogs in their "chlorophylled" ponds…

What about a relaxing hot bath? … The high temperatures in your bubble-filled getaway will draw even more water out of your body. However, as long as you account for the water loss, taking a hot bath will do more for your condition than worsen it. Outside of looking and smelling better, the embracing heat will calm your nerves and facilitate the release of more toxins. This is why saunas and steam rooms are so effective in the detoxification process... They make you sweat out toxins and chemicals... FYI: A spiked hot tub party is probably the most H2O robbing event you could attend (alcohol + heat + chlorine = 3x the dehydrating effects).

Quality H2O
In the U.S. tap water is definitely sanitary, but it does still contain traces of lead, chlorine, and other questionable substances... You don't have to be a professional on the molecular dynamics of H2O like Bobby Bouchet, but you should be aware that certain water sources are cleaner than others... (Yes, this means you *and* fido need to stay out of the toilet)!

Distilled water
This really is one of the purest forms available, but please don't go ransacking the chemistry labs for this taste... a gallon costs about a buck at the local store. Keep a jug handy in your dorm room.

Bottled water
Pulled anywhere from mountain springs or reverse osmosis factories, bottled water is available everywhere now... Statistics reveal that people are more apt to drink water if it comes in a bottle. Plus, most brands conveniently print the quantity on the labels so you can gage how much you're consuming. Stock up... If booze is affordable, so is water!

Filter pitcher/Faucet mount:
These are available in most stores...Keep a pitcher in your dorm room or if you live in a place with a kitchen, screw a filter on to your faucet. Certain brands actually have a mini "viewing window" revealing the contaminants being pulled out of the tap...

Hydrating foods
The following foods are high in water concentration and contribute to your daily intake: *Water*melon, pears, celery, grapes, tomatoes,

and of course cucumbers! … *not* pickles.

Pure H2O is best but most *<u>decaffeinated</u> and *<u>sugar-free</u> beverages *do* count as part of you daily water intake: Milk, juice, tea, soda etc…

*Limit beverages containing artificial and synthetic sweeteners. They are laden with toxins. Your better off sweetening your drinks with honey or other natural ingredients.

Bet you're ready for a few remedies
No… don't start cracking em' open again. "Haring the dog" just prolongs the agony! Don't you always feel worse after a weekend of partying than just one lush evening?
The following recommendations are known to dramatically reduce your symptoms:

Stop the Pain
Pop the ibuprofen or Tylenol. Both make headaches more bearable and reduce inflammation. Now if you're using these remedies practically everyday in order to get rid of a hangover, not a good idea! In high quantities the over-the-counters will inhibit liver function, and doesn't alcohol damage the liver also? Yes, in the long term taking too many coupled with alcohol abuse may contribute to poor health. Aspirin works also, but may contribute to the nausea… unless you have an iron stomach, you're better off with the following:

Certain foods contain natural pain killers
Delicious! According to Jean Carper's <u>Foods that Heal</u>, specific foods host salicylates (a.k.a. nature's aspirin). Not only do these foods possess anti-inflammatory properties and promote blood clarity… they help to alleviate pain with out the negative side effects of medication. (8)

*Your pain-reducing snacks include…
    -Apples
    -Cherries
    -Berries

-All peppers
-Almonds

*Please don't *O.D.* on these foods. Remember... everything in moderation! Nuts may be high in nutrients, but they are also high in fat.

Headache relief
Certain foods contain magnesium, a mineral effective for relaxing blood vessels... hence reducing headaches. (9)

-Whole wheat
-Leafy green Vegetables

*Curb the jitters with nature's sedatives
There are certain foods that aid to restore the natural GABA levels. Remember people have survived and slept well for centuries without the aid of drugs or alcohol. (10)

-Potatoes
-Mushrooms
-Rice
-Ginger
-Corn
-Spearmint

*Just like the "natural painkillers," do not *O.D.* on these foods either... everything in moderation.

Chamomile Tea
The noteworthy medicinal plant is extremely effective for calming nerves and promoting a restful night sleep. Globally used, this herb contains antioxidant flavonoids which help to fight free-radicals, protect against disease, and promotes an overall healthy immune system. It is available in most stores or anywhere tea is sold. Chamomile is naturally caffeine free and *alkaline forming throughout the brain and body... Drink it! Plus, it counts as part of

your daily water quota.(11)

*Maintaining an alkaline state is extremely important for optimal health and will be discussed in the next chapter.

Relieve an upset stomach or nausea
Primarily you need put food in your stomach, but don't overeat. Oversupplying the body with food of any kind will cause the stomach to produce more acid. The following are effective for absorbing and/ or neutralizing stomach acid: (12)

> -Bananas
> -Ginger
> -Plain rice
> -Corn
> *Whole wheat bread

*Try to replace *all* white flours and pastas with whole wheat... it contains fiber which pulls toxins out of the body.

Foods that may prolong a hangover and should avoid...
If you choose to consume "fast food," don't let it be greasy cheese burgers & fries, or a pizza loaded with sausage. Anything high in saturated fat is extremely acidic and will contribute to the inflammation. The negative mental effects of these foods will be discussed in the next chapter, but in terms of a hangover... well they really won't help your brain function any better. They also may contribute to existing nausea.

Fructose not glucose... This means the natural sugar in fruit is beneficial for your toxin filled body, but not the sugar in a glazed doughnut. If you are shaky or "withdrawn" the fatty baker's dozen may increase your symptoms. Besides, ingesting sugar is one of the fastest ways to ignite free radical damage.

Having a cup of coffee in the A.M. can help you kick-start your brain, but stop after one. Consuming caffeinated beverages as we know can be very dehydrating, and will contribute to the discomfort of your jittery neurological state.

Processed meats and other foods containing sodium nitrate or monosodium glutamate (MSG) may contribute to an existing headache.... as will skipping meals all together. (13)

*Other pain enhancing foods include...

> -Greasy fried foods
> -Mayonnaise, margarine, or butter
> -Sugary snacks
> -Pancakes (w/sugary syrup)
> -Heavy cheeses
> -Potato chips
> -Ice cream
> -Candy

*If these are the only foods available, then eat a small portion and try to avoid them for the next few days.

Vitamins/Herbs

Holistic medicine has certainly earned its place in society today, where astounding revelations have occurred. I do support most avenues of medical advancement as long as the intent is to genuinely heal people. Outside of a daily multivitamin and the following medically supported anti-hangover remedies, I will not be recommending diet pills or supplements in this book. I will however recognize the essentials within specific foods (in both chapters 3 & 4).

The following two remedies are globally recognized and highly recommended for reversing and preventing alcohol related damage...

1. **Vitamin C** – The C should stand for Chief because this vitamin is one of the most powerful Anti-Oxidants in existence, and is utilized as a natural remedy for almost everything. According to medical research,

appoximately 20 cigarettes alone will deplete 40% of the of the body's Vitamin C. Drinking alcohol will deplete it even further. Do your body a favor and take it!

2.   **Milk Thistle** – The herb protects the liver by making cells less permeable to toxins (i.e. your booze intake) and other pollutants by providing protection against free-radical damage.   It stimulates the production of new liver cells, while protecting the gallbladder and kidneys.   It protects the immune system while significantly reducing inflammation. (14)

This herb has poor water solubility so we need to ingest it through concentrated capsule form. Steeped teas are available, but not as effective…

*WORK OUT!

Of course this topic is a chapter in and of itself, but if anything gets rid of hangover symptoms, it's certainly exercise! It expedites the recovery process by:

1. Sending oxygen to the brain will help to remove the foggy sensation.

2. It increases oxygen levels and expels toxins from the body at a much faster rate (gets rid of the hangover sooner). The lungs are naturally responsible for eliminating the CO_2 (remember chimneys?). An increased heart rate will force O_2 into the lungs and into the bloodstream. This process coupled with an increased heart rate will clarify your system!

3. Increasing lymphatic drainage…Physical activity (especially jogging) will stimulate the lymph system, sending toxic waste into the bloodstream, which in turn exits though perspiring and urination.

4. Stimulating movement within the Kidneys, Intestines, and

bowel… yes, working out will send you running to the restroom… kicking out toxins at a quicker rate!

5. Creating endorphins… the brain's natural pain-killers

    *Remember to drink water!!

HANGOVER PREVENTION STRATEGIES

1. If you know there is going to be an alcohol-filled event… That morning start chugging the water. By around 5 p.m. you should have the majority of your water quota filled.
2. Consume high fiber nutrient-rich antioxidant meals that are low in fat, especially right before going out (see chapter 4 for dietary recommendations).
3. Avoid smoke-filled places… or don't stay there too long.
4. Avoid alcohol high in congeners: Brandy, Whiskey, Red Wine, and Heavy Beers
5. Drink water (or other caffeine-free & alcohol-free beverages) between cocktails
6. Take multi-vitamin in the early afternoon, Vitamin C (500 mg in the morning and 500 mg before bed) & Milk Thistle (200 mg. in the morning and another 200 mg. before bed)

CHAPTER 4

EATING... TO BECOME SMARTER & HEALTHIER

Your dietary chapter discusses: 1. Foods that hinder and hurt the brain 2. Foods that strengthen the brain by increasing attention span, enhancing memory, alleviating depression, and yes, increasing your I.Q. score... all of which promote a higher GPA. 3. Which foods keep us healthy (anti-oxidants/boosting the immune system) 4. The cleansing and detoxifying foods (fiber/chelation) 5. The importance of acidic vs. alkaline

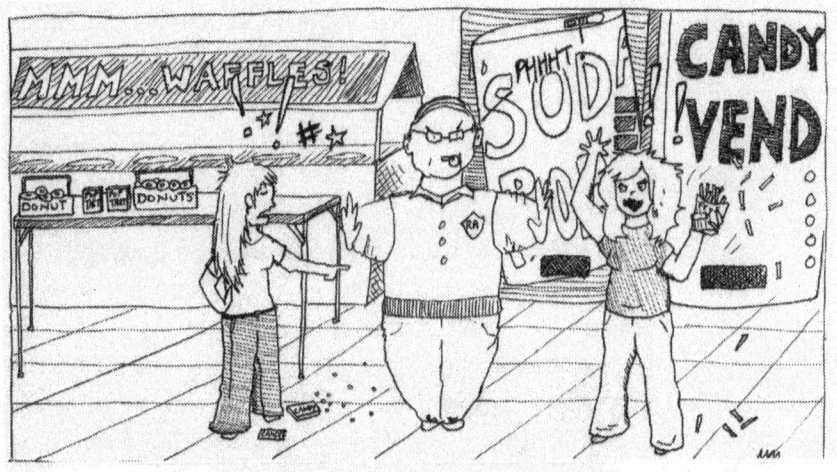

The back ground table (where they *were* sharing breakfast together) has a box of Pop Tarts, a six pack of powdered doughnuts, and two diet colas.

"You are totally bipolar."   *"Fine, then you soooo have ADD!"*

Wow, this cartoon is pretty darn accurate! Today we sling mental disorders around like they're four-letter words... think about it. How many times have we called someone a psycho, accused a foe of needing Prozac, or insisted that a friend was plagued with depression? Didn't people just used to say, "He's nuts?" Now we all deem ourselves psycho-therapists worthy of diagnosing the neighborhood… without script pads!

As a society we have become a bit "crazed" with craziness to the point where only a select few have remained unscathed of the loony branding. Not to disregard the need for mental health professionals or disrespect their jobs, but I bet you nine times out of ten, if you were to stroll into a shrink's office crying or wound up, they would peg you to be manic, have some level of anxiety, or at least be "temporarily depressed."

That kid down the hall you refer to as spastic is most likely sugar-sensitive and how about the countless number of women diagnosed with post-partum depression? Do you really think that there are *that many* new mothers out there bummed about their babies? Come on, not to enter the world of hormone replacement therapy… frankly I don't care to join the crucified line-up with Barry Bonds, but hello?… conditions such as post-partum are related to progesterone levels crashing and sleep deprivation, not the arrival of a beautiful infant (1).

Thank goodness for the M.D.s out there who realize a good portion of these "mental illnesses" are attributed to other factors including hormonal fluctuation or a malfunction in our food… not our brains! So before you start assuming your roommate needs Lithium or Ritalin, let's first get a clear picture of how the brain functions. Then we can take a look at what we're eating or not eating enough of. Remember, many of these "disorders" didn't surface until recently.

Understanding How We Think and Learn (how our brain retains and stores information)

Attention span, conceptualization, and memory are all primary brain functions (a relationship between the cells, neurotransmitters, and approximately 30 trillion synapses/nerve linkages). Dr. Mel Levine, M.D., one of America's top learning experts, shares that every brain is like a toolbox filled with delicate instruments. Our minds possess clusters of neurodevelopmental functions or a set of tools to learn each specific skill. For instance, one cluster may allow a person to comprehend and apply mathematical equations, another will enable an individual to memorize and recite the Pledge of Allegiance, while a third provides us with the capability of riding a bicycle. (2)

There are three categories of memory function, all vital components for academic achievement: *Short term memory* – used for very brief retention; usually about 2 seconds of new information. *Active working memory*- temporarily holds in mind all of the different components of what you are trying to do at that moment. *Long term memory* functions as the warehouse for permanent knowledge. This is where the storing of names, phone numbers, important facts, and the proper spelling of words is retained (3). The brain is an extremely complex organ that is affected by *anything* and *everything* we put into our mouths. Certain foods enhance the brain, while others can literally hinder its function!

"In fact, much more memory is needed for school success than is required in virtually any career." –Mel Levine, M.D.

<u>Foods (and other substances) That Hinder and Hurt the Brain</u>

MENTAL MALADIES
The following will inhibit healthy brain functioning (i.e. cause depressive symptoms, decrease attention span & memory).

Smoking cigarettes Time to attack the chimneys again. Tobacco triggers the release of cortisol (the stress hormone), which in turn lowers serotonin levels. This neurotransmitter is crucial for maintaining emotional stability.(4)

Drinking too much alcohol We have pretty much covered the negative ramifications of booze, including how it kills brain cells. This "brain damage" will inhibit your memory, attention span, and overall ability to concentrate. Excessive alcohol consumption is notorious for depleting B vitamins (mainly Folic Acid, Thymine, Riboflavin, B6, and B12), essential for warding off depression and enhancing memory. (5) And one more time, alcohol is a *depressant*! If you are in a depressed emotional state, drinking will worsen your condition… "Beer Tears."

Greasy/Fatty Foods: *(mainly trans fats or transfatty acids such as partially hydrogenated oils and other saturated fats present in some dairy products, poultry skin, red meat, baking fats, margarine, and butter)*

Yes, this includes your favorite pepperoni pizza, fast food french fries, cookies, milkshakes, and other great tasting, fat-filled goodies. Unfortunately these fats are considered to be "anti-nutrients" notorious for causing weight gain, stifling health, and inhibiting mental function. Numerous laboratory reports reveal that consuming bad fats will literally trigger inflammation resulting in a decline of brain function. It stunts mental growth, causes cognitive impairment, and memory loss! Small quantities are relatively insignificant, but definitely try to decrease your consumption of these foods (6).

Foreign chemicals in food…
There are over 2,000 unpronounceable fillers placed into our foods today (i.e. ethoxyquin, polyvinyl chloride, propylene glycol, MSG, and the list goes on)…. mainly to enhance appearance and taste, or to prevent spoilage. They are hidden in processed meats, packaged food products (instant meals in boxes or cans) or sprayed onto our produce.(7)

According to The A.D.D. and A.D.H.D. Diet!, most food additives/ preservatives are extremely harmful to the body. They deplete our immune systems and trigger behavioral problems (mainly ADD/ ADHD). Try your best to eliminate these foreign substances by thoroughly washing fruits and vegetables, aiming to consume foods with the *least* number of ingredients listed on the box, (8) and canning the Chef Boyardee!

Sugar/bleached flour/excessive caffeine
Certain mood disorders (anxiety, ADD/ADHD) are attributed to an over-consumption of sugar (glucose), bleached white flour, and caffeine. The troublesome trio literally robs the body of vitamins and minerals necessary for vital brain functioning. Meanwhile every medical source within arms reach reveals that an over-abundance of glucose in the blood stream will damage cells throughout the body. Sugar and flour in particular will create an insulin glucose imbalance leading to jittery rage-like behavior. (9)

Foods That Strengthen the Brain

Daily vitamins and minerals
Make sure you are fulfilling the standard RDA (Recommended Daily Allowance) by taking a daily multivitamin and incorporating foods in your diet that contain the following: Magnesium, Iron, Sulfur, Potassium, Phosphorous, Boron, Folic Acid, Vitamins B12, B6, Beta Carotine, Thiamine (B1), Riboflavin (B2), Zinc, Choline, Niacin, Chromium, Pantothenic acid, Coenzyme Q10, Glutathione, Lipioc Acid, Vitamins A, C, E, and Omega-3 fatty acids (good fats). There are many other beneficial nutrients worthy of mention, but these are the most important. (10)

Besides, we're not here to get dredged into a full fledged neuro-science course. Instead this book is here to be a fun and helpful resource for you, not a dry textbook demanding memorization. You have enough school work already…

So just like the hangover reducing food remedies … do not O.D. on these daily "vitals." Everything in moderation! For instance, Vitamin A and Zinc are excellent for immune function, but can pose toxic effects if consumed to excess.(11) At the same time cooking with olive oil is extremely beneficial for physical health and mood stabilization, but you don't want to gulp down five cups of it either or else it will cause weight gain. Always maintain your balance.

Briefly, before we get into the cafeteria food lines or venture down the grocery aisles, let's talk about the Omega-3 fats. No, they're not a newly chartered overweight fraternity with three members, but these EFA's (essential fatty acids) pose miraculous health benefits.(12) "What you ask... fatty acids? I'll get fat." Trust me you're more likely to be one of the three founders if you consume fat-free foods than if you solely consume the O-3's.

Manufacturers dump a load of sugar into fat-free foods to compensate for flavor-enhancing fat that they have taken out. The sugar-enhanced product is a recipe for mood swings and weight gain. O-3's on the other hand promote mental clarity and if consumed in moderation, will promote weight loss. (13)

Omega-3's are important for both our immune systems and mental health. Just like the body is comprised, if you want to enhance positive brain communication and proper functioning, you have to speak and communicate in the unknown "fatty language." And since the body cannot produce EFA's by itself, this means you need to ingest them through food sources or supplements.

Reducing depressive symptoms
Laboratory analyses reveal that depressed people are frequently deficient in Folic acid, Omega-3 fatty acids, and Vitamin B12. (14)To avoid being "down and out," up your intake of these three nutrients in particular:

Foods rich in Folic acid
Orange Juice
Avocados
Beans/Legumes
Oats/Barley

Foods containing Omega-3 fatty acids
Fish
Nuts (almonds and peanuts)
Seeds (mainly flaxseed)

Olives/Olive oil

B12 Foods
Eggs
Soy beans/Soy products
Seafood
*Milk/Dairy products

5-Hydroxytrypyophan hosted in lean meats and poultry is also beneficial for elevating moods: It helps to synthesize serotonin thereby reducing depression.
*Keep the dairy low/non-fat.

Increasing attention span, memory and your IQ!!

All B Vitamins
Across the board all B's have positive effects on the brain (Folic acid, B1 Thymine, B2 Riboflavin, B3 Niacin, B5 Pantothenic acid, B6 Pridoxine, B12 Cyanocobalamin). They curb mood disorders, revitalize memory, relieve anxiety, decrease depression, and promote mental focusing. (15)

> "Grape nuts... No grapes. No nuts. What's up with that?" –Cliff Clavin, "CHEERS!"

Put the "real" in your cereals...
Back to our balance... We would all love to pump in a canister of Captain Crunch or pretend oranges and apples are the true ingredients hosted in Fruit Loops, but they rank right up there with candy. Don't start eating junky cereals in college just because your parents wouldn't buy them growing up. If you were stuck with boring, low sugar Corn Flakes or Rice Krispies remember this: The only thing your parents "deprived" you of was toxic sugar. Thank them for keeping nutrients in your diet and investing in your "Jack in the box" ... and not "ADHD in a box." Most cereals and oatmeal are highly concentrated and are a great source of B Vitamins.

B1 Thymine: Optimizes cognitive activity and brain function: Brown rice, eggs, fish, peanuts, poultry, whole grains, broccoli, oatmeal, plums, prunes, raisins, & chamomile tea.

B2 Riboflavin: Aids to metabolize the amino acid Tryptophan which promotes serotonin in the brain: Eggs, fish, lean meats and poultry, spinach, whole grains, yogurt, asparagus, avocados, broccoli, mushrooms (not deep fried), leafy green vegetables, low/non-fat milk and cheese.

B3 Niacin: A memory enhancer and frequently used in the treatment of mental disorders: Broccoli, carrots, eggs, fish, lean pork, potatoes, tomatoes, peanuts, low/non-fat milk.

B5 Pantothenic acid: "The anti-stress vitamin": Eggs, legumes/beans, mushrooms, nuts, lean beef and pork, saltwater fish, whole wheat and rye.

B6 Pridoxine: Alleviates water retention, promotes normal brain functioning and RNA DNA synthesis in cells: Eggs, lean chicken & beef, carrots, brown rice, avocado, beans, spinach, peas, soy beans, corn, walnuts, sunflower seeds, broccoli, potatoes, cabbage, and cantaloupe.

B12 Cyanocobalamin: Prevents anemia, nerve damage, memory loss, and curbs depression: Eggs, seafood, soybeans, low/non-fat milk and dairy products (16)

Vitamin C contributes to an even higher I.Q. Score!
Remember? Outside of a daily multi, Vitamin C is one of the two supplements recommended in this book. Here's more evidence that this chief anti-oxidant is a miracle for the body: according to global consensus, an adequate amount of the vitamin will help keep students shoot above a "C" average. Scientific research unveils that IQ scores were significantly higher (5-10 points) in those students whose blood hosted higher concentrations of Vitamin C. Kids also scored higher on the test after incorporating orange juice (rich in

Vitamin C) for approximately six months into their diets (17).

Green Tea is loaded with polyphenols, special plant compounds that keep brain neurons healthy and blood vessels elastic so that nutrients can flow to the brain. The tea has been proven to enhance memory, alertness, and improve attention span. (18)

WHOLE GRAINS

Not to confuse them with common white flour and white rice, which convert into simple sugars or empty carbohydrates... whole grains are *complexed* carbohydrates. They contain three of the essential B Vitamins important for brain energy: Folic acid, B6, and B12. Great sources include: Whole wheat pasta, barley, oatmeal, brown rice and various whole grain breads. (19)

Nutrient rich and fiber filled choices...
-All Bran cereals, Kashi, Corn Flakes, Special-K, Rice Krispies, and others low in sugar quantities... Read the side label: (For example Rice Krispies contains 3g of sugar vs. Fruit Loops which contains approx. 13 grams)

PROTEIN

Consuming an adequate amount of protein will aid in the building and repair of individual cells throughout the body. This includes brain cells. As you know, cigarette smoke, dehydration, too much sugar, and foreign chemicals in our foods are the major culprits. Fortunately consuming moderate amounts of protein (always, always low in saturated fat) will help reverse the damage. (20) Now please don't go restricting yourself to a one of those carb-free, high protein diets. The body is not designed to handle only protein, for it over-taxes and damages the organs. Pretty much *anything* out of balance will ignite inflammation and cellular destruction. Great sources of protein are fish (best choice), *lean* meats, chicken, eggs, legumes/beans, and various forms of soy (be conscious of the fat concentration within these foods).

FISH

Fish has always been referred to as brain food mainly because of its high concentration of phosphorous. Phosphorous is important because it assists the body in the proper utilization of vitamins, and the conversion of food into energy. Fish is also high in zinc, which is important for immune function and protein synthesis. Additionally fish also has a high concentration of Omega-3 fatty acids. Our swimming friends will deliver an astronomical amount of thinking power to your body. Salmon, mackerel, tuna steaks (or canned in water/not vegetable oil), herring, menhaden and sardines are the best sources of Omega-3's in fish. (21)

CHOLINE

This amino acid has been scientifically proven and globally recognized to build strong brains and to maintain healthy brain cells throughout life. The FDA requires infant formulas (made with either cow's milk or soy) to contain choline. It helps to breakdown homocysteine, a harmful brain toxin. Choline is a precursor (building block) for acetylcholine, the neurotransmitter responsible for memory. Without choline, brain function and memory would become impaired. When people have Alzheimer's Disease, there is a severe malfunction within the acetylcholine transmitter. Great sources include: eggs, peanuts, fish, vegetables (mainly broccoli, cauliflower, and cabbage), low/non-fat milk and cheese. (22)

Enter the land of fruit & nuts

Here's some "iron"y* for you... People refer to California satirically as "the land of fruits and nuts." From a nutritional perspective this line actually translates into "the land of health and brain power." The silicon in the "Silicon Valley" is vital for cerebral function (the part of the brain responsible for thinking and observing). (23) Some of the most difficult schools to get into are Stanford and the entire U.C. system throughout the golden state. According to Michael, a 58-year-old professor of communications in the Chicago-land area, "Eating 10-15 raw almonds per day has completely erased *any* and *all* of my memory concerns. I've tried hundreds of remedies, to the point where I consider my body to be a permanent laboratory... Trust me. Almonds increase brain power!"

*Iron is a mineral hosted in almonds, vital for a healthy immune system, energy production, and blood flow. Other great sources of iron include some fruits: dates, peaches, raisins, pears, dried prunes, avocados, green leafy veggies, eggs, fish, lean meats and chicken.

Silicon sources include: whole grains, brown rice, soybeans, leafy green veggies, bell peppers, and beets.

OK... We need to have some fun here... At this point in the research game, I have encountered over 200+ articles, book passages, and medical journals that convince us to eat fresh berries (mainly blueberries), and they are all pretty much right on. (24) But reading the same thing over and over can become redundant, and frankly boring after a while. To make it worse, each "author" acts like they were the one skipping through the forest stumbling upon God's greatest creation: the blueberry. Great, can I be the one who invented the baseball?

Better yet, I'm pulling for the gooseberry! Why? Because of Snow White, that's why. Outside of her bad outfit and "Cinderella" complex, I think she got a bad wrap. Come on think about it... after she escapes an attempted homicide and cleans up after seven midgets, she finishes the day by cheerfully baking homemade gooseberry pies? In a midget's kitchen? I don't even know where to find a gooseberry let alone how to cook one. Well girlfriend does...So, Hi Ho dough and sorry for your crusty day!

Okay, so instead of telling you once again that blueberries fight free radicals, I found a quote that took first prize in exciting wordplay entertainment. Here it is...

"Berries are rich in anthocyanin pigments and potent antioxidants that build a **protective shield around the brain,** guarding against aging and damage to the brain."

And you thought becoming the "bubble boy" was impossible... And maybe this is why helmet laws are "unnecessary" in some states...

Hey and if they were mandatory, wouldn't it be great if we could just hand the peace officer an empty basket of berries instead of squealing out 50 excuses? ..."See officer, I've got it on!"

Alright between exonerating Snow White and the berry fictitious helmet law, this was very... random, but there is a reason for this silly tangent! If you have just gutted through these painful jokes, you have plateaued to one of the most valuable "brain" lesions that's been pounded into mine (just kidding- lessons): There is far too much monotony, fear, and negativity in the world. If you so desire to "Carpe diem," and soar with the U.S.'s regal emblem: Step up, join the faculty of life and contribute. Not from a fear-based, but a love-based heart!

"Remember; don't ever let your poems become ordinary." –Robin Williams in "Dead Poets Society"

"**Spinach** is an antioxidant powerhouse, bursting with beta-carotene, vitamin C and folic acid that help to keep blood vessels healthy and brain nerve impulses working properly. The iron in spinach is important for getting oxygen to the brain and improving concentration." (25)

Cool. Sound legit to you? Let's leave this alone. Especially if it still contains E Coli! What a shame. I'm sure that both the spinach growers and the food administration will eventually redeem themselves, and everyone will be consuming this green favorite again! But doesn't this ediet quote sounds like what happened to Popeye after Bluto pushed him too far.

Let's add one thing to it: ... Isn't it interesting how the two were always competing and literally fighting over "Olive Oil?" Not to applaud frailty or insinuate that they liked her because she was thin, but she was the thinnest female cartoon character ever drawn and named after an essential "fatty" acid. Wouldn't you bet that this cartoon mastermind possessed some nutritional insight in terms of spinach and EFAs (olive oil)?

How many eggs to eat?
Before his spaghetti sauce and salad dressing days, Paul Newman also hosted the label Cool Hand Luke. Remember that famous line, "What we have here is a failure to communicate?" That quote is from the movie "Cool Hand Luke," starring Paul Newman. However in this book he aced not failed communication… He turned the most dubious and obstinate inmates into his best pals. Now that rises to Machiavellian brilliance! Perhaps it was because he ate 50 eggs in one sitting. Doubt it. Remember too much fat causes a foggy mind and if you've witnessed this picture, he did wind up sleeping "in the box" for an evening. Watch this movie!

Outside of Luke's overindulgence… is it me or does everything relevant to ideal brain power have a relation to eggs (Choline, B-Vitamins, iron, protein etc…)? The yolks are densely populated with vital nutrients, but each little round ball of wonder contains 5 grams of fat. The next chapter will cover fat grams, calories etc, but if you were to order a 3-egg omelet, that would be 15 grams of fat and that's if your skillet had zero traces of cooking fat and the dish contained no sautéed veggies or cheese. Solution? To obtain the great taste and nutritional value, use one whole egg and the rest, egg whites.

Ask the Doctor
According Dr. Bernard Jensen, renowned historical author and authority on nutritional healing, it is no coincidence that the common mood disorders of today can be significantly altered through dietary change. The doc boldly stated… that "There is NO therapy or drug in modern medicine that can rebuild tissue that has been damaged by disease or trauma. Food, however, possesses the capability to be our true weapon against disease and illness." (26)

I love how Jensen chooses to term the foods he recommends as "healthful" instead of "healthy." The word healthful encourages a person to eat well, while removing the stigma of having to eat like rabbit in order to restore health or lose weight.

Meanwhile, other theories suggest that food allergies and sensitivities literally cause the brain to malfunction or swell resulting in psychiatric disorders... (27) Sounds like women aren't the only ones retaining water and many of the pros are proving our successful new balance to be true... A diet filled with ice cream sundaes *will* cause road rage. Don't you find it strange that the nuts on top are the ingredients keeping you sane?

Studying literally makes us smarter

Activities that involve thinking, learning, or undivided concentration will expand brain function. The brain doesn't actually grow larger, it become more efficient. Exercising the brain by thinking will literally switch on dendrites, synapses, and the overall effectiveness of the memory and comprehension (28).

Stress damages the brain

Short bursts of stress are proven to be beneficial for improving memory and overall brain functioning. However, prolonged periods of stress commonly brought upon by academic pressure, financial worries, or relationship problems will erode the brain resulting in forgetfulness. Research suggests that chronic stress will cause the hippocampus (the memory center of the brain) to literally shrink (29).

Physical Exercise Improves Brain Function

Exercise does a world of good for your mind! Outside of alleviating headaches, it causes brain cells to produce and expand. Infinite studies reveal that people who exercised 3-4 times a week scored significantly higher on tests that those who did not (30).

STUDYING TIPS:

1. *Right before bed is a crucial time... long term memory storage of information works best if you go right to sleep. You are more likely to retain test materials if you go directly to sleep after studying it. Do not start picking up the phone or go next door to visit with your neighbor. Don't take our "successful balance" out of context, but eliminate unnecessary distractions, and then dive into the*

material.

2. *Ask yourself this question: During study time, are you paying attention to what needs to be learned, or are you just going through the motions? If you are paying attention to what is supposed to be memorized... great. However, if the information is in one ear and out the other, you are wasting your time! This has now become an attention issue not a memory concern.*

3. *A great way to remember information is to transform it. For instance, if it's visual, change it into verbal. If it's verbal, make visual charts or graphs.*

4. *Write everything out. By writing on note cards, paraphrasing concepts from text books, or rewriting class notes makes information stick in the long term memory bank. Underlining and highlighting are also helpful.*

5. *Choose your study buddies wisely... Are they distracting you? Are they contributing to your attention static?... or are they allowing you to concentrate? You know.(31)*

6. *Read or study any class related notes/materials, or books during a workout. It will help your brain retain it more effectively!*

The ancient C.R. "Diet"
"In general, mankind, since the improvement of cookery, eats twice as much as nature requires." –Ben Franklin

Although a bit chubby, Mr. Franklin certainly had a way with the pen (I mean feathered quill) and was one of our nation's most brilliant diplomatic inventors. The C.R. stands for Caloric Restriction, and the "diet" is more of a guideline. This doesn't translate into skipping meals... please don't. The theory behind this is not only for weight loss and aiding to avoid the "freshman 15,"... it *promotes brain functioning, and boosts the immune system!*

How? Why? Food digestion is considered to be high maintenance on the body. Immediately after we consume a meal, our bodies naturally go to work for us. Our metabolic system breaks down the heavy proteins, fibers and carbohydrates. Then regardless of what we're eating, our bodies have to sift through and differentiate between the true nutrients and foreign toxins.

This process alone requires the undivided attention of our immune systems to fight off the chemicals and bacteria hidden in our foods. In fact, people who overeat or are constantly stuffing their faces, either develop illnesses faster or do not live as long.

Unless you have been advised by a doctor, I do not recommend going on any fad diets… statistics reveal that in the long run, 90% of diets fail! So outside of routine exercise, a balanced C.R. diet, and simply following the food pyramid printed in numerous health books and everyday food labels (more of this in Ch. 5), don't diet. Eventually your cravings will catch up with you.

Envision it: A long week of dieting (or deprivation) and then Friday night rolls around. You decide to blow off some steam with friends, indulge in some lower calorie cocktails, and 1:00 am rolls around and your buddies start the pizza orders. I'm sorry but if you are even remotely under the influence, when that delivery boy arrives, goodbye diet! If you hadn't deprived yourself all week long, the pizza cravings wouldn't be so strong. Boom, wake up Saturday morning and its guilt time. Then you start the diet again, put in a monster workout yadda yadda, and the cycle begins again. Obviously no one is perfect and of course slip-ups (binge eating) are inevitable, but if you just eat moderately the majority of the time, then these "food swings" are less likely to occur.

Which Foods Keep Us Healthy?

Boost Immune System

I know, it's the antioxidants again coming to the rescue by stopping free-radicals dead in their tracks. The antioxidants in fact work on the cellular level, not as an entire shield. They possess special compounds that can donate an electron to the unstable molecules without become unstable themselves. This act of giving will allow cells to live longer. There are a number of <u>vitamins</u>, minerals, and other phytonutrients that act as powerful antioxidants, working to neutralize free-radicals and protect healthy cells. Glutathione, beta carotine, vitamins A, C, and E, selenium, <u>carotenoids</u>, flavonoids, and alpha-lipoic acid are all potent antioxidants.

Antioxidants are mainly found in plant foods, fruits and vegetables including: all berries, carrots, broccoli, kiwi, spinach, tomatoes, red peppers, bell peppers, watermelon (NOT IN JUNGLE JUICE), prunes, citrus fruits, avocado, and sweet potatoes.

The Miraculous powers of garlic
Yes this one is hubbed in Cali also and displays one of the best festivals of the year. In their modest home, the proud people of Gilroy, California offer everything from garlic bread, to garlic fries, and even garlic ice cream? Why make such a big deal over garlic? Well for centuries these little bulbs have been used for medicinal purposes; mainly because they host sulfur. Sulfer helps reduce liver damage, kills bacteria, literally halts tumor growth, prevents weight gain, prevents the common cold, and reduces overall inflammation… Eat it!

<u>Cleansing/Detoxifying foods</u>
Both high fiber and chelating foods literally possess the ability to directly excrete toxins throughout the body by binding them and pulling the waste out of the body!

One doctor went as far as comparing the effectiveness of chelating foods to "like swallowing a bottle of liquid Drano! That's how well these foods purify our bodies (foot Born)." Fiber is essential for the removal of toxins, but also is essential for weight loss (More in Ch 5.)...

Chelating foods
Carrots, apples, bananas, seaweed, alfalfa sprouts, garlic, onions, fiber-rich cereals, beetroot, and watercress

High fiber foods
Whole fruits and vegetables, whole grains (breads and cereals), brown rice, and legumes/beans.

The Importance of Acid Vs. Alkaline Foods

AVOID Acid-Forming Foods: Many of the foods we eat create an acidic PH balance which sparks inflammation and internal free radicalization throughout the body. This is a common breeding ground for both brain deterioration and illness. Acid-forming foods include: 1). Foods that are processed, containing preservatives, added sugars, fillers and lectin-filled flour products 2). The second type of acidic food includes added hormones and hydrogenated fats. 3). The third group of acid forming foods host caffeine, and alcohol. Others include: potato chips canned/sugary fruits, milk (cow) cocoa, and red meat.

CONSUME MORE Alkaline-Producing Foods: These foods promote calming-like effects through balancing insulin-glucose levels and curbing inflammation. This in turn will promote healthy functioning of the thymus gland and a higher production of T-Cells. Not only does this stabilize the entire immune system, it encourages cellular renewal within all connective tissues (tendons and ligaments), blood, fat and skin cells in the body.

The alkaline-forming good carbohydrates include brown rice, buckwheat, and most legumes or beans. The alkaline-forming good fats include the omega-3 fatty acids, flaxseed oil, and soy.

Beverages that counteract the acidic state are: some herbal teas (sage, green, mint, and chamomile), buttermilk and water. The vegetables include: asparagus, celery, and broccoli. The Fruits: apricots, cherries, apples, figs. The nuts include: mainly almonds and sesame seeds. The dairy: yogurt. The herbs are: basil, ginger, and pepper.

CHAPTER 5

YOUR MEAL PLAN (PART II)
ELIMINATE THE FRESHMAN 15!

This chapter addresses weight gain in relation to the foods we eat: 1. Are you overweight? Check it out by measuring your B.M.I. (Body Mass Index)

2. What are calories and how many to eat per day? ... 3. The Secrets for achieving Metabolic Balance with your meal plan, The Sugar impact, The truth about carbohydrates, Slimming fiber, How many fat grams per day? And... more water! 3. The importance of breakfast and why it's important to choose foods lower on the Glycemic Index 4. The power of protein 5. What else is keeping the weight on? 6. Eating in social situations 7. More strategies that keep the weight off! 8. How to avoid emotional eating 9. Thinking yourself thin!

*"Don't worry even if things end up
a bit too heavy we'll all float on
all right"*

-Modest Mouse

Approximately 70% of the people in the United States are statistically overweight, while 50% are literally obese. Excess weight boosts the chances of heart disease, diabetes and even cancer... why? Too much fat hosted in the body is unhealthy. Remember where the body stores toxins? Both deep within the lymphatic system and individual

fat cells!

Check your BMI
If you *are* concerned that your weight may be becoming a problem, a simple way to check it out is by calculating your Body Mass Index (BMI) and then comparing your value to the everyday recommendations. Now please do not take your BMI number to heart! This is just a basic "ballpark" of where you're at.

*To calculate BMI:
1) Multiply your weight in pounds x 704.5
2) Divide the result by your height in inches.
3) Divide the result from step two by your height in inches, again.

The result will be your BMI. Unless you are an athlete with lots of extra muscle, the following applies (muscle mass is more dense than fat):

Underweight: Below 18.5
Low weight: 18.5-24.99
Normal/Average: 25.0-29.99
Overweight: 30.0-39.99
Obese 40.0 or more

The difference between being overweight and being obese is: overweight people possess excess muscle, bone, fat, and water relative to height. A person who is obese hosts an abnormally high proportion of body fat…

If you are content with your body weight and appearance, great! But for those of us who are "self dissatisfied" and roll our eyes at the thought of bathing suit weather, the following advice will help…

First, you need to maintain an accurate food log for one week… It sounds tedious, but if you aren't accountable for what you're putting into your mouth, how can we truthfully assess your situation? By the way, 99% of us only really require a slight alteration, not an entire transformation of our eating habits!

"To thine own self be true"
One of the main reasons people gain weight is not because of body chemistry or having the "fat gene." … It's because folks are not being honest about their daily food and beverage intake (i.e. excess fats, sugars, & carbohydrates). Generally speaking, I've found that people are either oblivious or in denial of what they are putting in their mouths!

As a personal trainer, I can't tell you how many times I've listened to clients complain about their weight, and all the while swearing up and down that their diets are completely free of "fattening foods." Extremely frustrated with the lack of results, they always ask "How can I get this weight off?"

And the same advice is always relayed: "OK people, if you are working out as much as you say you are: incorporating weights, cardio and strength training… and you're <u>sure</u> the doctor said your thyroid is operational, than the culprit is most likely the diet!" On just about every occasion people are either eating/drinking too much, or too much of the wrong things.

There's one lady who sounds like broken record saying, "I'm so fat…. My boyfriend and I had pizza again last night. Oh well, I must be getting my period." For the first few weeks this excuse was acceptable where I thought maybe she just had an extremely irregular cycle. But after six months of listening and adding up the inflated PMS stories, she was averaging three periods per month, and two late night pepperoni pizzas per week… after dinner! And every time I asked to see her diet log, "Oh I forgot again. I'm just too busy to do it." Then of course as the following training session would approach, she'd roll in with the same sob story *again*… "Help me I'm getting so fat…"

This is the definition of insanity, people. Doing the same thing over and over and expecting a different result. If you are in this type of cycle, please read <u>Who Moved My Cheese</u>? It will bring you a lot of insight into life and the patterns you choose to live by. Similar to this book, it is a quick and easy read.

If you want to make progress with your physique, it's time to start looking in the mirror. Yes sizing up any undesirable waist lines and saddle bags is certainly relevant, but even more important... look into your own eyes! You can fib to family members, friends or a personal trainer, but is it possible to lie to yourself? Only you know whether you've devoured that entire bag of Ruffles or exceeded your daily allotment of calories in any way. Come on, you can't eat five calorically dense bagels in a day and expect to not gain a pound (even if there is only one gram of fat per bagel). It still equates to approximately 1,600 calories. By the way "calorically" is not a word, but it made the sentence flow... so we begged the editor to leave it in. Why not? I'm not hurting anyone's feelings; just describing a bagel.

Moving forward!
Great, now that everybody is accountable and learning blatant disregard for the English language, let's start incorporating some nutritional science. Wait! Don't turn the book into a hockey puck just yet! This may sound bland, but many of the recommended foods are full of... not sugar, but flavor & and spice! Understand that your body is extremely complex and therefore requires *some* empirical explanation. Several factors contribute to weight gain/weight loss, but let's try to simplify this as much as possible.

How many calories am I allowed per day?
Loaded question... Factors such as existing muscle mass, the amount of cardiovascular exercise/weight training you engage in, and your metabolic state certainly dictate this number... but to give you a rough idea... (1)

*Between the ages of 18-21
Males: 2,400 calories per day
Females: 1,800 calories per day

*This calculation is based upon those who exercise less than 30 minutes per day

Now a general rule, any calories burned (i.e. through working out) may be added back into your daily allotment. So if you burned 300 extra calories by speed walking, than you may carefully add 300 more calories into your diet… It's a basic math equation. Now when we discuss weight training/muscle building in the workout chapter, you will be able to add even more calories to your daily amount.

Yea… Back to the Booze!
Just a brief reminder in case you skipped the section on "The caloric values of your cocktails" in Chapter 2…

1	12 oz.	Beer	=	Approx 140 calories
1	5 oz.	White wine	=	Approx. 90 calories
1	1.5 oz.	Rum/Vodka	=	Approx. 97 calories
1	1.5 oz.	Liquor	=	Approx. 155 calories

Calories add up quickly! Going out on a Friday night after consuming breakfast, lunch, and dinner? … Your 5 beers can add up to 600-700 calories alone. And we wonder why freshmen gain fifteen pounds? Now if drinking was part of your high school career, so many other factors were keeping the weight off: Mainly Sports, eating high quality meals at home, and other calorie burning activities that kept your metabolism high. Now it's all about the heavy/fried foods in the cafeteria, late night greasy pizzas, beer, and no sports: AKA the recipe for a slower metabolism and packing on the freshman 15!

Don't forget to add in the Mixers!
Remember when you're calculating the caloric total of a mixed beverage to not only add the calories from booze, but to incorporate the juice, daiquiri mix, sugary slirpy, or whatever you're dumping into the booze.

One 8 oz. serving of juice, regular soda, or mix will add an average of *115-155 calories* to your beverages…

Achieving Metabolic Balance

The metabolism is your body's engine... or the chemical process through which living cells assimilate food. Metabolism is simply defined as the number of calories you are burning at any given moment. So when we ask the question "How many calories should I eat in a day?," the key to your answer is revealed through your daily allotment of food (calories, fats, & carbohydrates), exercise/physical activities, and the amount of muscle mass hosted in the body. Ideally you want to keep your metabolism revving in a higher gear to keep the weight off. The following are seven major factors that control your metabolic rate (for the better and worse).

1. What you eat and drink (quality)
2. How much food you eat (quantity)
3. When you eat
4. Water consumption
5. Amount of sleep/cortisol levels
6. Cardiovascular exercise
7. Your muscle mass

Numbers 6 and 7 will be covered in chapter eight, but the following will cover 1-5...

AVOID EATING TOO MUCH SUGAR

Oh it's in there alright... sugars are hidden in so many of our everyday food products (snacks, spaghetti sauces, canned fruits & veggies, and of course baked goods). Don't boycott Hawaii, but consuming excess sugar will definitely contribute to weight gain. Today the daily recommended allowance is 12 teaspoons of sugar per day on a 2,200-calorie diet, but the U.S. Department of Agriculture discovered the norm to be 31 teaspoons out of a 2000 calorie diet. Cut back by reading food and beverage labels (2). Sugar causes insulin levels to spike signalling the body to store more fat!

Finally...more truth about Carbohydrates!
Carbohydrates are actually made up of thousands of glucose molecules, which upon digestion are converted into individual glucose molecules. The glucose is released into the bloodstream and

then becomes "fuel" for the body. Any excess glucose that has not been burned up completely is stored in the liver and various muscle groups... Once their reservoirs are filled, then the glucose is converted into fat and deposited into adipose (fatty tissue).... Cellulite. This explains why carb-free diets have gained such popularity. The over-consumption of carbs (mainly sugar, refined and starches) will convert into fat storage. (3)

As a fitness professional, I will NEVER recommend going on a "diet" at all let alone any faddy carbohydrate restricted diets. There are just too many vital nutrients hosted in carbs to deprive the body of them (i.e. fruit, whole grains etc...).

Which foods are Carbs? Primarily, carbohydrates are in grain-type products (i.e. bread, pasta, flour, rice, and baked goods). Potatoes and corn, along with most fruits and vegetables fall within the carb circle as do many of our beverages (mainly sugary juices, sweet wines, darker beers, liquors, and cordials).

"Refined" grains (another form of "empty" calories): Refined means that close to if not all of the nutrients (vitamins, minerals, & fiber) have been removed from the food product either to enhance flavor or to increase shelf life. Examples include white flour, "non whole wheat" breads, bagels, pastas, tortillas, crackers, buns, and rolls. "White" rice is also categorized as refined as are most cereals. However manufacturers will "fortify" cereals, by adding iron, B-Vitamins, and bran to compensate for the refining process and to replenish some of the nutritional value.(4)

"Whole" grains: Whole means that the grain or food product is unaltered, or still hosts all of its nutritional value (fiber, vitamins and minerals). Whole grains are found in oatmeal, popcorn, brown rice, and breads/pasta/rolls/tortillas/buns that have the word "whole" in product: i.e. "whole wheat bread" or "whole grain pasta." Many food labels will read "100% wheat bread." This can still mean that the bread has been baked with "refined" wheat flour. The label has to say "whole" in order for it to be legitimately unrefined. (5)

Why is it so important to eat more whole and less refined? Because unrefined "whole" products are not only healthier for you, they help keep the weight off! How? 1. "Whole" grains contribute to a feeling of fullness causing calming food cravings, preventing overeating. 2. Whole grains boost metabolism because they are filled with *fiber, thereby taking a longer time to digest and absorb. 3. White flour and other "refined" carbs contribute to blood sugar imbalances. When too much glucose is released into the bloodstream (caused by ingesting too much sugar and other refined carbs), the body reacts by releasing an overabundance of insulin. When too much insulin is present... the body thinks you are in "survival mode," hence signaling fat storage. Contrarily, whole grains are released slowly into the bloodstream and therefore do not convert as quickly into glucose. This in turn controls insulin levels which inhibits fat storage.

*Fiber: Yea! Nature's most powerful diuretic! In both soluble and insoluble forms, fiber is applauded for: 1. Filling you up, hence the prevention of overeating 2. Works as an internal scouring pad cleansing your organs and removing toxins stored throughout the body. Great sources of fiber include: Whole fruits & berries (Not the juice. It contains sugar and the fiber is strained out), Grapefruit, oranges, grapes, apples, blueberries etc... and most vegetables: carrots, celery, bell peppers, cucumbers, and all the leafy greens etc... and of course "whole" grains.

Fiber aids in weight loss?

Yes... Countless medical professionals theorize that weight gain may be attributed to an abundance of microbiota (the bacteria hosted in the gastrointestinal tract). And a significant amount of this G.I. accumulation is attributed to consuming inflammatory foods such as: Sugar, starchy refined carbohydrates, and unhealthy fats (mainly in red meat). (6) Antioxidants certainly aid in damage repair, but fiber cleanses and rids the G.I. tract of the microbiota bacteria. This contributes to weight loss!

Potato Skins (extremely high in fiber): Not to start a cookbook here, but one of the most nutritious fiber-enriched meals can be created from a potato... Not the ones served as appetizers at the local food chains! Ouch, loaded with starch and lard. Some campus cafeterias have potato bars. So grab a hot one in or out of the foil, scoop out 1/3 of the insides, and refill it with all kinds of healthful foods over at the salad bar. Get creative, but don't go drowning it in ranch dressing!

Instant fiber

Instant soups, not to be confused with "cup-o-noodles." More so black bean and lentil soups are excellent sources of fiber and a healthy part of a balanced meal... They contain only 200 calories, 10 grams of fiber, 9 grams of protein, and only 1 gram of fat per serving.

Follow the Glycemic Index

One of the body's primary challenges is to maintain an intricate balance between glucose and insulin. Essential for providing nourishment to the entire system, their operative balance is crucial moment to moment (Too much insulin results in hypoglycemia, where a dominance of glucose induces a "sugar high"). The two work in conjunction transporting fuel to the core (mitochondria) of the cells. Their system controls the appetite, cravings, and weight gain. This active pendulum remains balanced when we ingest foods containing healthy fibers, proteins, and moderate amounts of glucose (mid to low on the glycemic index).

The glycemic index is a ranking of carbohydrates based on their immediate effect on blood glucose or blood sugar levels. It compares foods gram for gram in exact measurements. Carbohydrates that break down quickly during digestion (sugar and refined grains) have the highest glycemic indexes. The blood glucose response is fast and high. Foods that break down slowly, releasing glucose gradually into the blood stream, are ranked lower on the glycemic indexes. Glucose and Insulin are a function of one another: When blood sugars are high, the body naturally secretes counteractive insulin. Consequently when insulin levels are dominant, the body cries for sugar (glucose) to obtain balance again. (7)

Any inner conflict existing between insulin and glucose will lead to turmoil within the bloodstream. This in turn prompts insulin to signal the release of cortisol (the stress hormone) and the body to store fuel as fat (weight gain).

Consume more foods lower on the glycemic index (slow to convert into glucose sugar):

- Melons (cantaloupe, watermelon)
- Green Vegetables (spinach, broccoli, and asparagus... not peas)
- Plums/Peaches/Pears
- Citrus Fruits (oranges, grapefruit, lemons)
- All Berries (don't forget gooseberries)
- Lean Meats (chicken, lean beef, pork, turkey)
- Beans/Lentils
- All Fish
- Hummus
- Lettuce (all types)

Avoid those high of the glycemic index (they convert into sugar too quickly):

- All candy
- White flour (hosted in pancakes, waffles, pastries, doughnuts, or baked goods)
- Most crackers and *sugary* cereals (i.e. frosted flakes and fruit loops)
- White rice and rice cakes
- Sugary/Starchy vegetables (corn, peas)

Condiments

Hey I love BBQ sauce, relish, and ketchup as much as the next person... Definitely lower in fat, but notorious for hosting ...a lot of sugar. Use sparingly and try to substitute ketchup and BBQ sauce with salsa or mustard. Baked beans are also loaded with sugar.

Ketchup   1 Tablespoon contains 4 grams of sugar
Baked Beans   ¼ Cup contains 12 grams of sugar

FATS

Good Fats: We covered the healthful importance of EFA's and the Omega-3's in chapter 4, mainly in fish, avocado, olive oil, and flax seed oil.

Bad Fats: Outside of inhibiting brain function, in higher quantities they contribute to weight gain. "Bad fats" are the Trans-fats/saturated fats hosted in meat, poultry skin, dairy products, coconut oil, and palm oil.

Obviously you want to consume more "good" fat, but too much of anything will prompt a nasty reaction. Just like calories, a daily allowance of fat exists: (8)

Males: 18-30 years old 6 tsp. of fat per day (approx. 24 grams of fat).
Females: 18-30 years old 6 tsp. of fat per day (approx. 24 grams of fat).

Foods that quickly drain your daily allotment: (9)
1 doughnut 18 grams of fat
1 piece of cake 16 grams of fat
1 small bag of potato chips 11 grams of fat
1 cup of whole milk 8 grams of fat/ 1 cup of 2% milk 5 grams of fat
1 small order of fast food fries 27 grams of fat

The times a "fat free" label is better
If you've ever baked or watched someone bake a cake or cookies from scratch, one of the main ingredients outside of white flour, is sugar. Doughnuts, cookies, cakes and other baked goods are loaded with it! If you're going to eat these sugary foods (please in small quantities),

you're better off choosing the fat-free cake over regular cake. You might as well remove the excess Crisco or vegetable oil. Besides, many of these non-fat recipes are made with healthy applesauce or fruit juice to compensate for the lack of vegetable oil. Fat-free baked goods are not necessarily good for you, but are certainly the lesser of two evils! Also, definitely choose fat-free milk over whole milk or even 2%.

FYI: An average raised yeast doughnut contains 8 to 12 grams of fat. A single cake doughnut can have up to 22 grams of fat. Besides the calories, doughnuts can pack a hefty dose of unhealthy saturated and trans fats ("bad" fats). Remember, your saturated fat effects the hormone insulin… by eating too much saturated fat we develop insulin resistance… it becomes less efficient at handling blood glucose levels… weight gain.

Our bodies crave healthier foods
While serving in the National Guard, they required us to attend monthly meetings where doughnuts and coffee were served religiously. Month after month, jelly-filled, chocolate, glazed you name it. So one morning I decided to conduct a little experiment by purchasing a few dozen semi-ripe bananas and putting them up against the routine morning "goodies." By the time the meeting was adjourned, over half of the doughnuts were still in the box, but *ALL* of the bananas were eaten. Why? Follow me over to the…

Tailgaters & Parties
No coppers following into this paragraph (you're supposed to be avoiding doughnut shops anyway). Let's talk about the fun Saturday pre-game and post mid-term celebrations. The N.C.A.A. may just have a dual meaning (No Cops Allowed Anytime)! Definitely collegiate perks and places where the best foods are! We all love BBQ's and all of their side dishes. Every time I've ever attended or hosted a function where food is served, guess which foods are eaten first? Most people select the grilled chicken and fish over a greasy cheeseburger… and the vibrantly colored vegetable and fruit salad dishes (not the hot pink icing drizzled onto doughnuts) are usually

chosen over the macaroni salad drowned in mayonnaise.

Protein
Speaking of fish and chicken, nothing keeps a body more toned than lean sources of protein. After participating in multiple body building competitions this an arena where I host authority: Knowing how to exercise nutritional discipline… There were countless mornings where I've wanted to dive into Aunt Jemima's sugary cap, knowing all the while a lean, protein-filled breakfast represented a win.

Why is protein so effective for maintaining weight loss?
Protein takes a lot longer to digest than carbohydrates, hence promoting appetite suppression. Similar to whole grains and fiber, foods higher in protein take a lot longer to digest and enter the blood stream. This in turn reduces insulin and overall fat storage.

Secondly, hemoglobin, the blood's oxygen carrying molecule of the blood is built from protein, vital for cellular existence: Proteins break down into amino acids, which repair and strengthen individual cells (including muscle tissue)…. The more muscle mass we host, the more fat is burned. This will give you that lean, toned and flab-free appearance.

Eat in moderation
Not many people can stomach an all protein diet anyway, but if you've become part of this rarity, definitely be careful… protein in high quantities can certainly overtax and place additional stress on the organs (mainly the liver and kidneys). (10)

Preferred protein sources include:
      Lean beef and pork*
      Skinless chicken breasts (chicken wings are extremely high in fat)
      Fish: Salmon, tuna, (try to avoid breaded or fried)
      Shellfish (shrimp, lobster, crab)
      Nuts and seeds
      Legumes, beans

> Many whole grain products
> Low/non-fat dairy (milk, cheese, & yogurt)
> Eggs (one egg yolk per meal & the rest whites)

*Avoid greasy bacon, white ribbed steaks, and hamburger exceeding 10% fat.

What time are you eating?

Eating late at night will put the weight on! It's quite simple: As we progress into the resting hours our ability to burn calories slows down. I find the "Don't eat after 6:00 p.m." rule is a bit strict… unless of course you're going into surgery the next morning, where late night fasting is crucial. Smaller low/non-fat bedtime snacks are fine, but avoid eating large meals late in the evening. Aim to place your heaviest load of calories during the earlier hours of the day which brings us to one of the golden rules in weight loss…**Eat breakfast!** Almost all nutritional experts agree that eating in the morning boosts metabolism and promotes weight loss. Consume foods that are rich in protein, higher in fiber, and low in fat: Oatmeal, cereal w/ skim milk, fruit…

Eat before you exercise

Eating before a workout will increase your energy levels allowing you to exert more effort, hence burning more calories. Besides I always like to provide clients with a kind forewarning: Please get a decent night's rest and definitely eat something prior to your session. I don't come right out and say, "I will be kicking your a—tomorrow, be ready," but the majority comprehend the underlying message. Don't forget to wait at least twenty minutes after you eat before starting to exercise.

Overall, I recommend a correlation between a reasonable diet, exercise and following the basic food pyramid. Eat fiber-rich whole grain carbohydrates, fruits and vegetables, lean protein, and choose healthy fats. Of course watch your caloric intake and get plenty of physical activity.

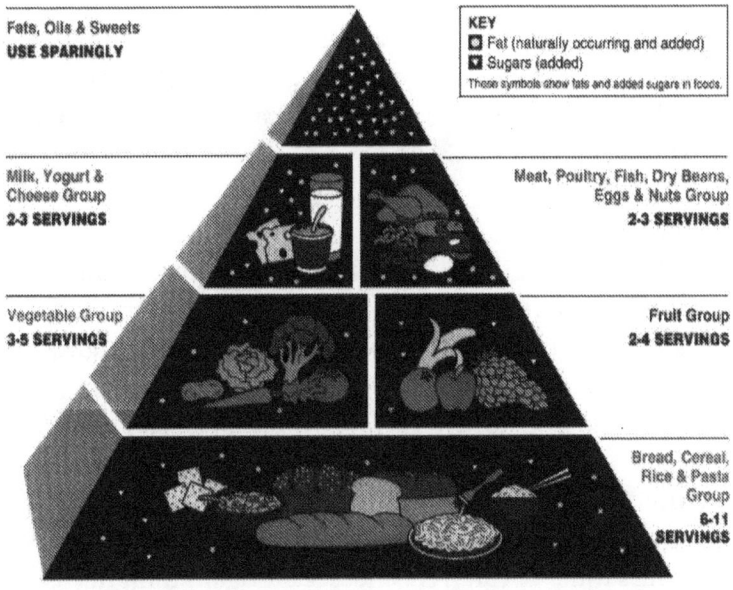

Diagram 5.1

MORE REASONS THE WEIGHT STAYS ON...
NOT EATING ENOUGH

By not consuming enough calories in a day, we are telling our metabolism to SLOW DOWN! The body is trying conserve to keep you alive. Slashing too many calories, particular protein calories, pushes the body to conserve calories rather than burn them. It also forces your body to break down muscle tissue to fuel its vital operations. But that muscle is the key to your metabolism, or the speed at which you burn calories. More muscle promotes a faster metabolism and less body fat.

Waiting until you're famished to start eating... or eating too fast

Remember it takes the brain 20 minutes to register from feeling hungry to feeling full. So if you find yourself gobbling down a huge plate of pasta or an entire pizza for dinner without stopping, you're probably eating so fast that your stomach hardly has time to alert your brain to tell your mouth to quit chewing. Then after 20 minutes, your stomach feels like it's going to explode. This means you've consumed too many calories, fat grams, carbs in one sitting… great way to gain weight.

Lack of sleep

When we sleep less than seven-eight hours per night, it ignites cortisol and raises insulin levels… which in turn stores fat! Chapter 1 discusses strategies for achieving a more successful night's rest.

Falsified workouts/Believing: "As long I work out I can eat whatever I want!

How many people have we seen in the gym spending half of their "2 hour workout" socializing by the water cooler? "Oh I worked out for two hours today; I can have cheesecake again tonight!" OK great, but how many calories did you actually burn? Also, a twenty minute stroll on the treadmill at 3.0 MPH will NOT earn you that extra 600 calorie dessert in the cafeteria "sundae bar!" It's a basic math equation. We cannot eat more than we burn off.

Too much stress

Stress raises cortisol, which in turn causes insulin to become dominant in the body. This causes the body to store fat.

Not drinking enough water

When we are trying to lose body fat, proper hydration is essential. You need it to flush the waste products your body makes when it breaks down fat for energy, or when it processes protein. You need it to transport nutrients to your muscles. It aids in digestion and the upkeep of a higher metabolism.

Let's meet for coffee

Are you ordering coffee or a double shot extra foam vanilla mocha surprise with whipped cream… and sprinkles on top? Uh doesn't this sound familiar? Kind of like the ice cream sundaes we agreed in chapter 1 that should be kept as a secondary reward… Coffee drinks are perceived as low in calories, but over the past couple of decades coffee houses have managed to doll up your java drinks to rank up in fat and calories with Baskin Robbins. FYI: One 16 oz. mocha (hot or iced) hosts 347 calories, 16 grams of fat, 41 carbohydrates, & 28 grams of sugar... and this is made with only 2% milk. What about the alternative low-fat coffee coolers? Definitely a lot lower in fat (3 grams of fat in one 16 oz. beverage), but contains 40 grams of sugar, 48 carbohydrates, and 230 calories.(11)

Now get back in line with your pal or study buddy... Order just coffee or tea and if you need to add sweetener or milk, use 2% or skim if you can stand it, and a packet of splenda. Stills needs more flavor? Add cinnamon. This magic spice not only tastes great in coffee, it's an ancient remedy for curbing appetite.

Turn your pizza into a healthy meal!
Order thin or whole wheat crust, half the cheese, skip the fattening toppings like pepperoni and sausage... instead top it with fresh bell peppers, mushrooms, garlic, onion, or chicken... When it arrives on your plate, use a napkin to dab off any signs of grease...This ordering method will save you loads of fat grams and calories... If your friends ask why you're ordering so healthy? Tell them, "I read this is a new way to order pizza and salad at the same time."

My friends will make fun of me if I avoid fattening foods
Most guys won't notice if you snack on a few peanuts or have just one slice of pizza while you're out, but ladies tend to be very conscious of who's eating what. We'll address these annoying social issues within the individual gender chapters, but in terms of coping with catty social eating situations: 1.Eat before you go out. 2. Eat what's there in moderate quantities, but remember to tread lighter the next day. 3. I'm not saying you need to change your group of friends, but you may want to incorporate some health-conscious pals into your life... But make sure that it doesn't turn into a competition over weight loss or a sabotaging beauty contest... Try to help each other!

MORE TIPS:

Eat smaller meals more frequently Many of us (especially those who've served in the military) are conditioned to eat three square meals daily. Try to disperse your food consumption by eating 4-5 smaller meals throughout the day. This in turn will eliminate dips in blood sugar levels while preventing an excess of insulin release (fat storage).

Great snack ideas include whole and dried fruit, low/non-fat yogurt, whole wheat pretzels, crackers, popcorn, dried and whole fruit, low fat string cheese, nuts, fruit and vegetables.

Drink water

"We suck again!" –Rob Schneider "The Water Boy"

Consuming an 8oz. glass of water before and between meals is extremely effective for curbing appetite. And definitely hydrate before, during, and after you exercise, as it is essential for successful weight loss. Our bodies are made up of approximately 70% water and without it, weight gain and fat storage are inevitable. It's fascinating to know that nine times out of 10 when we are "hungry" grabbing for food, what we really are is thirsty. High quality H2O is also an important component of any serious weight-loss plan. Since thirst is commonly mistaken for hunger, remaining hydrated will keep you from overeating. (12)

Emotional snacking
Okay, you fell out of a tree and what did mom do? Outside of applying a Snoopy band aid, she handed you a cookie. How about those all-around bad days? How did we celebrate the pain… perhaps with the best of Ben & Jerry? Now by the time you've stopped falling out of trees or started falling in love, how old are you? Some start falling in love with trees, but regardless of the growth scenario, approximately 80% of our brain's programming has been established… and so has your emotional association with food.

Now What?

Great news! Remember this: It only takes 3 WEEKS to change or instill a new habit. See and we didn't even have to get Freudian about this! Just revert back to the Doctor in chapter 1... Yes, delicious Dr. Suess and all of the places we'll have to go in life. But this doc never mentioned hitting the doughnut shop when you're down and out. And he allotted to perhaps winding up on a deserted island not hitting the dessert aisle.

Developing a Thinner Attitude towards Food
Have you ever taken notice to the behavior of "naturally thin or fit" people? You know the people who have "perfect bodies" without even trying. Yep, the girl at the BBQ eating the cheeseburger twice her size... Meanwhile you're easily 10 pounds heavier and holding a tiny bowl of fat-free pretzels chirping in a pal's ear, "That is so unfair. She's so skinny. I can't remember the last time I've even looked at anything fattening, let alone put it in my mouth." To make it worse... She's not even thinking twice about the grease that's practically dripping down her arm. Better yet she looks so happy! How? Why? Well, after following a couple of skinny people around for five plus days, here are a few of their truthful "tails":

1. They lead positive & stable lives
Don't things seem to just go right for these people? They appear to be virtually problem free ... But the reality is they are handed a plate of life's choices and upheavals just like you... They carry heavy class loads, yet seem to persevere regardless of the curriculum level. Their expectations are realistic and almost always possess futuristically balanced attitudes. Their moods are relatively serene, and they handle stress quite well.

2. They don't obsess over food
Unless required, naturally thin people aren't preoccupied with how many slices of turkey are on their sandwich or whether there might be an extra squirt of mayonnaise on the roll. They eat a fraction of meals and do not find it necessary to clean their plates. They eat slowly and food is a SECONDARY issue on their minds.

3. *They aren't obsessed with weight*

Thinner people could really care less about what *anybody's* weight is, let alone their own. Perhaps they have an innate trust that their bodies will regulate themselves. Whatever the reason, you won't see thinner people jumping on a scale first thing in the morning…
Final Notes:

During public lectures, I love sharing the "5 Golden Rules to Better Health" with an audience:
1. Drink ½ your weight in water daily as discussed in chapter 3
2. Incorporate exercise (chapter 8)
3. Eat breakfast every day
4. Increase your consumption of fruits and Vegetables
5. Minimize **C.R.A.P**

    Caffeine
    Refined sugar
    Alcohol
    Processed foods

More happy endings:

1. Follow the basic daily food guidelines (i.e. allotment of calories, fat, fiber and protein)
2. If your jeans are getting too tight, don't just throw them away or blame the new dormitory drier for their shrinkage… be truthful about your diet and alter it accordingly (consuming the proper quality and quantity of foods & drinks, times to eat, and of course when not to…)
3. Don't obsess over food. Ask yourself this question: "Are you living to eat or eating to live? Aim for the latter!

CHAPTER 6

THE COLLEGE LADY

Your chapter discusses social issues during the college years: 1. Dating advice... Where guys' heads are at and where their priorities lay 2. How to tell the good dates from the bad 3. Safety and appropriate conduct 4. What type of women gentlemen are trying to avoid (Cinderella Complex/MRS Degrees) and which ones they're looking to date (the balanced modern lady of today) 6. The effects of alcohol on the female body 7. Stress and Hormones in relation to weight gain 8. Understanding how and why your body may have changed (less tone and the development of cellulite mainly in the hip, thigh and butt regions...)

"I never realized until lately that women were supposed to be the inferior sex."
–Katherine Hepburn

"This one's for the girls."
-Martina McBride

Helmer: Remember-before all else you are a wife and a mother.
Nora: I don't believe that anymore. I believe that before all else I am a human being, just as you are."
-Henrik Ibsen

Dating in college
Let's kick off your chapter by talking about boys. We'll get this discussion out of the way because it's a heated topic and frankly hooking up with guys should fall short on your list of collegiate priorities. "WHAT? You have got to be kidding right? WHY," you ask? ... I'm not saying don't date. Just keep those boys as secondary

desserts. Remember the overly gratified kids of today we discussed in chapter 1? Well the same thing applies here. Both school and establishing true friendships should be the most important to you now. Allow me to explain.

What's in his head?
Well first of all males enter college primarily to receive an education and of course a vast percentage of them are there to party. Now whether they join fraternal organizations, compete in intramural sports, or frankly do nothing but go to class.... The one thing *all* college guys agree upon is this: "We are not here to get married!"

During these years (ages 18-22), males feel a social obligation to first become established in life (i.e. earning a degree and finding a stable career) before they even consider settling down and having a family. This doesn't mean guys are repelled by committed relationships, but just don't expect a matrimonial ceremony in the middle of your university union.

Okay, now let's get to the sticky topic of males in this age group. Their sex drive is at its peak and guess who they're eyeballing? Yes, you. Now don't develop the attitude that all guys want from you is sex. Try to be objective and comprehend it as a natural physical reaction. For instance, when a heterosexual male sees your cleavage through a revealing blouse, nine times out of ten, he will become aroused... to the point where his pulse literally goes up! Men are very visual beings. It's their biological make-up. Don't panic! This doesn't mean that men are completely incapable of exercising fidelity. Remember your eyes drift also...and as they should, but within reason!

Alright this brings us to everybody's least favorite ancient gender battle: "Men staring at other women." It sparks arguments at parties, bars, and would probably even arise at a funeral! It happens in all age groups throughout the globe. Right now there's probably some lady in Tibet reprimanding her guy for eyeballing the neighbor's daughter...On and on and on!

Enough! Too much wasted energy. There are two quotes that fly out of my mouth during confrontational situations: 1. I don't do dramma (yes with the double m) and 2. My name's Paul and that's between ya 'all! Fighting is something that I avoid like the plague. So allow me to provide you with some peaceful armor upon entering this century-old jealousy arena... Now as we said *everybody* falls guilty of people watching whether we're madly in love with a certain someone or not.

But here's where the fine line needs to be drawn: Is he just glancing in passing maybe once or twice at another attractive woman? This is acceptable behavior and still within appropriate boundaries. Remember even *you* notice and admire another beautiful woman. However, if he is *really* looking to the point where it's chronic and he simply will not peel his eyes off of her... RED FLAG! If this blatant behavior is happening to you on a date, this probably indicates one of three things:

1. He's not committed to you or your relationship is not on solid ground (remember you are in college and he's not there to get married).
2. Nasty to hear but he probably wants to pursue the girl he's eying.
3. He's not a faithful guy/perhaps even a player. This means he's probably not the best candidate for dating. It's not that he won't be in the future, but certainly not now!

Ladies, the same aggravating stuff happens to guys on dates too, okay? I'm not trying to upset anyone. Instead I want you to be objective and to not own or internalize your date's behavior. Understanding and sifting through this crap will avoid countless brawls during your college days (especially if you've both been drinking). Now if you are being faced with a date from hell, follow this advice:

1. If you're angry (which you probably are) don't show it. Remain composed. Remember this is his obnoxious behavior not yours!

2. Don't start getting pissed at the girl he's eyeballing. She may just happen to be on her own date and not there to pick up on yours.

3. The most powerful thing you can do is walk away. That simple act will give you back so much power. Frankly, you'll probably make him feel like an ass… good for you!

4. If you're the strong brave type, start staring at other guys and give him a taste of his own meds! This could be comical, but be cautious that it might spark an argument. Still be prepared to walk away.

5. Take this as a blessing in disguise… He'll probably be a rat in the future! Hey at least it's socially acceptable for you to shed tears. Men possess plenty of emotion as well, but he's perceived as a wimp if he even thinks of welling up.

Whew! Glad that's over.…

Safety and Appropriate conduct
This brings us to the discussion of safety precautions. Guys are not necessarily a bunch of wolves, but unfortunately there is always going to be a predator out there somewhere. Being preventative and effective planning will dramatically reduce your risk of becoming a statistic. Now gentlemen should ALWAYS exercise self control and there is NEVER an excuse for a man to sexually violate a woman. If this has happened to you, it wasn't your fault! Call for help! The university clinics, RA's and of course the police are there for your protection!

Now some of this advice may seem repetitive or obvious to some, but your families truly worry about your safety while you're away at college… especially on those Friday and Saturday nights. So please follow these rules, okay?

1. Make sure you go out to parties with a girlfriend or where other females are present. Sororities have great buddy systems as do many residence halls.

2. If you choose to drink, gage your BAC level; see Chapter 2.

3. Don't sleep over at fraternity houses or where a house full of guys live (even if you are with a girlfriend).

4. If you're coming from the library late at night or you have evening classes, make sure someone walks with you. Most universities have shuttle/escort services… Use them!

5. Not here to rearrange your wardrobe or to tell you how to dress… But a fact is a fact: The more you reveal, the more they have to stare at! You can control that. This is a college campus not a beach. Got it?

6. Carry Mace!

What Guys don't want (Cinderella/MRS Degree)
Society has a tendency to program women to believe they need to land the right man. And that "right" man is generally strong, ambitious, from a good family, and of course holds a healthy wallet! Why, so he can rescue and take care of her for the rest of her life. La La la la la la la la and live happily ever after. Sound familiar? This is known as the universal epidemic: Cinderella Complex. This fairy foo foo tale completely contradicts why a female attends college. Just like guys, women are supposed to be there to earn a degree, graduate, and indulge in a career. A guy can sniff out a girl who wants to be taken care of a mile away… and unless they are the type of guy looking for the Barbie trophy wife they hate that needy bloodsucking behavior…. College guys refer to female huntresses as, "Those chicks looking for the MRS degree!"

What type of lady gentlemen are looking for
I'm sure the majority of you ladies are in college to get an education and strive for self reliance, not to just meet some guy. You are fully aware that 1955 is long gone and the responsibilities of men and women are changing. Women are playing vital roles in the workplace more so than ever before. Men are starting to share the spotlight. There is nothing more attractive to a man than a woman with goals and ambition. Yes ladies you like men with equal ambition, but trust me if you want to be successful in the dating world, you have to have a lifeline or something you want to do with your life.

Still want to be Cinderella?
Okay let's grab his wallet and the wand! Remember though… a princess never becomes overweight and looks perfect at all times. She doesn't drink beer or wouldn't even think of touching a cigarette! By the way I don't recall Cinderella ever macking out in the bushes with prince charming… that would be unheard of and so unladylike! Oh yes, and she most definitely makes it home before midnight! Awwww Are you ready to puke yet? Is it from the princess rules or maybe it's from the beer bonging competition earlier in evening? Dump the tiara, get your degree, and have fun! That's what will make you truly happy in the long run. Oh yeah, and guys like women who are happy.

All my friends are guys…NO
It's great to have a tomboy air coupled with some male friends, but it's so important to acknowledge and embrace sisterhood as well. By not befriending women, you're indirectly trashing your own gender. Too many male friends may make a potential sweetie edgy, and you don't want that getting in the way of a love interest. Do yourself a favor, be a *true* good friend to your girlfriends too. Besides when you do finally *truly* earn that MRS in front of your name (after your bachelor's), your male chums can't exactly be your bridesmaids!

In Oprah's *O Magazine*, January 2006 issue good ol' Dr. Phil relays some perfect advice of "seven qualities of women you want to be around:" His checklist is pretty constant to what guys are looking for in a girl…

1. *Women who see the strengths, not the limitations in others. They make you proud to be yourself-because they tell you why you're special.*

2. *They trust you so fully that you feel compelled to meet their expectations. Consequently they make you feel like a better person than you normally are.*

3. *They respect you for what you have done and where you have come from.*

4.   *They are authentic and don't need you to lie to them to feed their egos.*

5.   *They live by their rules but don't expect you to follow them.*

6.   *They are at peace with themselves, so they don't have to prove anything to you.*

7.   *They're good listeners and sincerely interested in you, so you feel important. Because they're available for honest and genuine discussion, they make you want to share yourself.*

If you notice, <u>never once</u> did Dr. Phil recommend wearing less clothing, "putting out more," acting like an airhead, or engraving the trendy "tramp stamp?" Yes that black jagged tattoo in the lower back that many younger women feel compelled to get these days. Instead, he talks to the relevance of women having integrity, being sincere, and maintaining their individuality.

Some more dating advice...

Should men always pay for a date? Easy. Let's not fall back into Cinderella mode. He should certainly pay if he asks you out. Now if you ask a guy out, you should pay. Done... Unless of course the two of you have a mutual "Dutch paying" agreement, this rule should apply and avoid disagreements.

How do you know whether a guy is out for "one thing?" If a guy truly likes you (wants more than just a fling), he is more likely to move slowly because he doesn't want to mess things up. He'll be the one initiating non-sleazy conversations and he'll probably be inquisitive of your personal life. He'll be genuinely interested in what you have to say! On the other hand if you're at a party and some cute "screw ball" is pawing at you all night, guess what he probably wants?

I really like this guy, should I play hard-to-get? No, but similar to what he's doing… move slowly and instill balance… Talk to him. Ask questions and care about what interests him, and most importantly be a good listener! Guys hate it when girls ramble on and on about themselves, or better yet… What ever you do, don't keep repeating yourself or relaying the same stories over and over! Now if he asks you out for a specific day, don't lie or pretend you're too busy for him. Be honest: If you have class that evening, don't say, "I'm busy that night." Tell him, "I have class that night." Or if you have a study group in the library at that time, ask if you can meet later that evening or the following day? Deception sucks! Plus it will only drive distance between you both.

Don't date more than one guy within the same fraternity, club, or workplace! Wait until the magic is truly there! Because contrary to popular opinion, guys often gossip… and a lot more than women do; and so sorry but some boys will be mean and TALK! TALK! TALK! …….. Trash yeah and trashing your reputation!

HAVE A LIFE!

Develop a genuine interest in your collegiate "career." Go to college for a solid reason outside of meeting guys and partying. Develop a core relationship with your major/classes and make friends. These things are more attractive to guys than your looks! Guys like girls who are interesting!

The effects of alcohol on the female body
First, women have lower total body water content than men of comparable size. After alcohol is consumed, it diffuses uniformly into all body water, both inside and outside cells. Because of their smaller quantity of body water, women achieve higher concentrations of alcohol in their blood than men after drinking equivalent amounts of alcohol (3). So be careful when chugging with the guys.

Outside of Chapter 3's graphic explanation of boozal detriment (another made-up word that sounds great); alcohol causes the liver to slow down the metabolization of estrogen in a woman's body (4).

In other words, drinking will cause women to possess too much estrogen.

Hormonal imbalance is never a good thing. Estrogen stimulates insulin and progesterone tempers it. Estrogen dominance leads to stress, anxiety, and the release of insulin (5)... Remember from Chapter 5 what happens when too much insulin is in the body? It signals the body to store fat and ignites cravings for sugary heavy carb foods. Excessive drinking will often cause menstrual disorders (e.g., painful menstruation, heavy flow, premenstrual discomfort, and irregular or absent cycles) (6).

Stress affecting your hormones/weight gain
Women possess three primary sex hormones: Estrogen, Testosterone and Progesterone. Between the ages of 18-22 they are generally heightened and balanced, hence being the ideal natural child-bearing years. Please listen, this is not a reason to go out and get pregnant! Don't worry you will have plenty of time to have babies. Female hormones remain heightened for decades.

When you stress out or become out of balance, so do your hormones. Stress inhibits the body from releasing progesterone posing the same estrogen dominance that alcohol consumption causes i.e. irritability, insulin floods, food cravings, and weight gain (7).

Obviously cutting back on alcohol and maintaining stress levels (working out Chapter 8) will certainly help your hormones to stay in balance. In addition, one professional Dr. Holly Lucille ND, RN suggests that the ideal avenue for maintaining balance is through controlling the way in which hormones are metabolized. Proper liver function is extremely beneficial, as is diindolylmethane (DIM) a powerful nutrient found in cruciferous vegetables such as broccoli and cauliflower. So according to Dr. Holly, eat these veggies ladies (8).

Why do I have cellulite and look flabby now?
Most ladies were relatively active in high school with sports and

other activities. This in addition to eating healthier at home helped you maintain your metabolism and toned figure. As you know life suddenly changes in college where you're not playing competitive sports and are now in control of your diet. More than 90 percent of women are affected by cellulite. This condition can be disfiguring and certainly affect your self esteem. There are many other factors that cause cellulite, including:

- Poor circulation
- Defective connective tissue
- Enlarged fat cells
- Poor diet and nutrition habits
- Lack of exercise

According www.mesotherapy.com, Dr. Lionel Bissoon explains that cellulite passes through three stages of cellulite. Stage 1: No visible cellulite when standing or lying down, however cellulite can be seen when skin pinched. Stage 2: Visible cellulite when standing, but not when lying down. Stage 3: Visible cellulite when standing and lying down. (9)

How does it form
Fat cells develop in the subcutaneous level and are arranged in chambers surrounded by connective tissue called *septae*. As water is retained, the fat becomes trapped within this area, expands and stretches, and eventually contracts and hardens (sclerosis) inhibiting flexibility of the skin. As the surrounding tissue continues to expand or weight and water gain continue, these areas of the skin continue to remain stagnant, while other sections bulge outward revealing cellulite.(10)

Why do women develop it but guys generally don't?
The body hosts receptors that either break down fat (Beta-receptors) or create fat (Alpha-receptors). Above the waistline, the number of alpha to beta-receptors generally equates to a 1:1 ratio in both males and females. However below the waist, women have approximately 6 to 8 alpha-receptors for every beta (high cellulite region). This is

the reason why women have difficulty losing weight in this area. Alpha-receptors (fat promoters) are generally stimulated by the consumption of carbohydrates, fats, amino acids, hormones, and alcohol (11).

Obviously the most effective way to eliminate cellulite is through diet, exercise, and drinking ample amounts of water, but cutting back on alcohol will definitely help dissolve it.

CHAPTER 7

THE COLLEGE GENTLEMAN

1. Dating in college: What are the girls looking for, and what they detest about men! 2. Avoiding Peter Pan & 7 common myths many guys believe about girls clarified 3. Safety, & appropriate conduct... i.e. controlling your hormones and frisky libido 4. Male competition: The Pressures to drink each other under the table 5. Safety in Fraternal life/Hazing 6. The negative effects of marijuana and alcohol on the male body (i.e. xenobiotics and testosterone converting into estrogen) 7. How and why guys develop "love handles" and "beer bellies"

"He won't sell anybody out to buy his future! And that, my friends, is called integrity. That's called courage. Now that's the stuff leaders should be made of. He's chosen the right path made of principle that leads to character. When the s--- hits the fan, some guys run... and some guys stay. Here's Charlie facin' the fire and there's George...hidin' in big daddy's pocket. Whoo-ah!"

-Al Pacino "Scent Of A Woman"

Dating in College
In the lady's chapter, we did our best to explain to them where your heads are at, the type of dates looking for, and of course the ones you're trying to avoid. Here we'll attempt the same for you.

What are girls looking for?
Well let's first get physical... No not literally! I'm talking about appearance.... Sorry I forgot for a second there that I was speaking

to an audience encompassed of 18-22 year old guys. Ladies would obviously prefer a gent who was easy on the eyes (nice-looking), but believe it or not most girls aren't gravitating towards bulging muscles either. Yeah no need for steroids! In fact nine times out of 10 women prefer a naturally toned and average natural looking body on a guy. A handsome face and great hair definitely fly higher on the priority list, as opposed to most of you who are willing to blow the whistle and settle for a million dollar body and a ten cent face.

Once past the physical… to most ladies, nothing is more attractive than a guy who's the B.M.O.C. (Big Man on Campus)… Yep, that notorious power thirsty female stereotype some girls can't seem to shake. And hopefully that "Who's Who B.S." will eventually diminish, but until then it exists. Just like there's a percentage of you only out to get laid, some girls are shallow and only want to be with powerful men. So look out if you're the president of the Inter-fraternal Council (IFC) or the heir of Bill Gates. Titles like that will definitely score you some chicks. But is the attraction for the right reasons? Are her feelings for you coming from deep within the heart? Well perhaps if she's gotten to know you extremely well, but most likely it's more of a crush or surface situation. Now if your fraternity gets thrown off campus or if Microsoft goes belly-up and she's still with you, then you got a keeper.

Okay, now the masses. In everyday situations, girls love guys who possess confidence, intellect and wit. I don't care who the chick is… they ALL love a guy who can make them laugh. But don't try too hard to play stand-up comic upstaging every other person in the room. It has to flow naturally. Trying to achieve the class clown title is not the objective. We've already gone over the physical criteria and a clown wasn't on the list; not even for Halloween dress up. Not appealing! If she's a psych major, she may try to break through to your inner child and use you as a case study for her midterm paper. NAAAAA. Just keep your silliness and comedy childlike, not childish!

Women Hate Cheating Peter Pan behavior!
You take 99.9999% of women and ask them if it bothers them if

you're scoping other chicks and they will say: "UGGG… That is the worst!" They hate (and I'm using the word hate because they feel so passionately about this) it when the guy they like is always interested in the next better looking woman who walks in the door. This is part of the universally titled Peter Pan complex! Girls become disgusted and aggravated if they perceive a guy just wants a one night stand. Women hate players! Have you ever seen the movie Fatal Attraction? Do not scorn a woman! Cut out the stringing along mimbo behavior…(1)

Don't worry guys, the ladies caught an earful about emulating Cinderella and were given a clear understanding of how much you loathe that deadweight "princess." They've been given effective strategies on how to shelf their tiaras. Anyway, back to you. The following are some tips of how to bring Peter out of NEVER land…

The ladies got advice from Dr. Phil and for you we have elected renowned relationship specialist (No not Dr. Ruth) Dr. Barbara De Angeles Ph.D. to discuss seven common myths that may help understand your lady friends better.

MORE? You want to get along with women, don't you????

The 7 Myths Men Believe about Women debunked! (2)

1. Women are never satisfied! False! The truth is that when women are with a man they truly adore, they are passionate and committed to making it work between the two of you. She's not dissatisfied with you; she just wants the relationship to be the best it can be.

2. Women are high maintenance. Nope, intimate relationships in general are high maintenance for everyone involved. If your lady appears to be requesting a great deal of communication from you, it means she's taking the time to care about your needs and interact positively with you.

3. Women just want to control men. Wrong again… Women want

to contribute, improve/help you, and be included in your life. They don't want to control you or prevent you from having a life. They want to enhance it.

4. Women are jealous and possessive... Nope. They're just being protective of their emotional highly valued relationship. They feel threatened if they feel you are being aroused by another female because it could potentially damage what you have between you.

5. Women are too emotional. Well let's just say women are in touch with their feelings. Girls are legendary for venting. Remember the majority of the time, they just want you to listen, not fix their problems.

6. Women who appear to be strong and competent don't need to be taken care of. Please try not to be intimidated by a strong or independent lady. They are not out to compete with you. They just have career interests and passion about life like you. Every human being wants to feel nurtured, loved, and have a partner they feel they can lean on. Even you! Besides, guess which ladies really need you most? The ones who are always strong and taking care of others.

7. Women want to rob men of their freedom. Wipe the "ball and chain" idea out of your mind! Women just want to create a committed intimate relationship, and to be included in your life. They aren't trying to isolate you from your friends, family or schoolwork/job.

Remember the Triple A's: Attention-Affection-Appreciation

Okay, now you know why they get upset when you appear interested in another woman, or exclude them from the tailgaters on Saturdays. If you don't want a committed relationship in college, that's fine. The fact that you are not at college to get married has been relayed to them in their chapter. Be respectful, truthful, and just draw boundaries if you don't want to fall in love and be committed. This information is definitely helpful once you do choose invest in a loving commitment.

SOME MORE DATING ADVICE...

Who should be paying for dates? Keep this simple. I know it's the traditional for the man to always pay a lady's way, but today there's a different set of rules. If a woman asks you out, she should be the one willing to pay the check. Now if you ask her out, you should pay. Done... Unless of course the two of you have a mutual "Dutch paying" agreement, this rule should apply and avoid disagreements.

How do you know if she's the Cinderella-Type? If a girl truly likes you (wants more than just cash or a status bump), she is more likely going to move slowly because she doesn't want to lose you. She'll ask you questions about your life, and how you feel about certain situations. A gold digger will be preoccupied with things like what your parents do or what neighborhood you grew up in. She'll find out whether you're on scholarship or not. She'll talk about money, who's rich that she knows, and of course frowning upon people who are poorer. The lady who's interested in you will be genuinely interested in what you have to say!

I really like this girl, should I play hard-to-get? No, but certainly don't ignore her. Approach the situation slowly, carefully, and instill balance... Talk to her. Ask questions and genuinely take interest in what she has to say. And most importantly be a good listener! Girls hate it when guys brag about themselves or discuss other women in attempt to make them jealous... Now if she asks you out for some occasion on a specific day, don't lie or pretend you're too busy for her. Be honest: If you have class that evening, don't say, "I'm busy that night." Tell her, "I have class that night." Or if you have a study group in the library at that time, ask if you can meet later that evening or the following day? Deception sucks! Plus it will only drive distance between you both.

Don't date more than one girl within the same sorority, club, or workplace! Wait until the magic is truly there! Because stories get around and you may become the topic of comparison... ouch! You don't want to be labeled a sleazy player. Don't trash your reputation!

Physiological sexual irony
Alright so eighteen is when males peak sexually, and college years are 18-22 so you are there buddy!! That's right, the more frequent erections and sexual urges. You've been placed into this scientific fertile bracket for a good reason: Procreation and to ensure the survival of the species. However, there's a bit of a discrepancy here if you haven't figured out because #1 I really doubt any of you guys are ready to be pushing baby strollers around campus. #2 it's ironic, for college is the time you are not supposed to get anyone pregnant. You have four (or five depending on your work ethic) years of studying, memorizing, and producing term papers.

Be careful with intimacy!
Women are a bit different today than say ten years ago.... Even in the winter, their clothes seem to get smaller and more revealing and sexually suggestive. Simultaneously a lot of women are consenting to following through what their outfits are offering. This is still an area where you need to be sooooooo careful! As we discussed in the girl's chapter, the more they reveal, the more the guys are going to eyeball. We explained that they have control over their wardrobe choices. However, no matter how sleazy she's dressed or acts, it does not grant you a true physical sexual invitation. Let me be frank: No means No! And if she's pushing you off... get off! And go get off somewhere else. Rape is a felony. Period. Right Don?

Drinking each other under the table/Male competition
The statistics are devastating with alcohol-related deaths on college campuses. I know how fun it can get with the Friday happy hour coupled with the Mexicali & quarters games flying! But, again please refer to the B.A.C. chart to gage your drinking! There's always going to be someone pushing the next painful yagermeister shot in front of

your face, "Come on…. What are you, a p---y?" You know the guy. If you know you've hit the ceiling in terms of the amount of booze you've already consumed, push it back and walk out!

Hey I'd rather be called names like that, than hit a BAC of 4.0 and wind up in the ER… hopefully! Check out of that scene. They probably won't even remember heckling you to drink anyway. If you do have friends (more like acquaintances) like the ones forcing you to drink heavy, duck out early, make excuses, or say you have to meet some chick. Of course changing your so-called pals is an option. But if anything, try to limit the "bar time" you spend with them.

Greek Organizations and other Clubs/Hazing

I believe whole heartedly in joining any organization or club that will enhance or strengthen a student's collegiate experience. Besides, close to all fraternities and sororities support the academic success of their members. They compete against the other houses quarterly or per semester for the highest GPA's on campus. They all want to be #1. Plus, they require a certain amount of library or in-house study hours, especially of those members whose grades are falling.

The pledges especially are kept on a short leash academically and to some degree treated with a parental tone throughout their pledge ship obviously to deter any out of control wild freshman behavior. Greeks are not necessarily all about partying. All houses participate in philanthropic events and most are quite strict on how each member conducts themselves. In fact, most of these organizations host internal disciplinary committees to maintain ethical, respectful, and responsible behavior.

Speaking of respectful, this now also brings us to ritual… Similar to many religions, Greek organizations host beautiful and authentic ceremonial traditions to maintain the sisterhood/brotherhood, while embracing and extending the spirit to new members… most rituals date back to the 1800s. Pretty cool…..

Hazing

Sometimes outside of ancient ritual, certain chapters will incorporate their own local traditions. Although usually meant well, these practices can sometimes involve excessive drinking or physical roughhousing…behavior that can ignite trouble. If you are a member of a Greek organization, you understand the bonding between a big/little brother/sister. It can be an extremely special experience, but don't get out of control with it. So before you start a drinking contest with your newly initiated little bro, check back to the BAC chart in chapter 2! There's a fine line between love and hate, but sorry death and alcohol poisoning are not part of brotherhood! Plus, don't you want to remember the bonding experience and have a little brother for that matter?

Smacking each other around? Yes boys love to rough house, but you never know when somebody's parent may get pissed off at you and your local rumbling ritual. Besides, what happens when you inflict physical harm upon a pledge (or anyone for that matter)? A.K.A. Assault and Battery! Yet another felony UG! BE CAREFULL!

Effects of alcohol on the male body
Not that you're attempting to reproduce at your age (get a girl pregnant), but excessive alcohol consumption can damage testicles and lower sperm quality for future offspring. As we discussed in chapter 2, drinking alcohol in excess will obstruct the liver's enzymatic activity, necessary for eliminating estrogen surplus. This has negative effects upon women, but for males as well. Heavy drinking promotes femininization (excessive estrogens) in males who are hormonally sensitive. A dominance of estrogen over testosterone is the recipe of demise for gentlemen. Estrogen excess not only leads to significant hair loss and gynecomastia (female-like enlarged breast tissue), but depression as well (3).

Effects of marijuana on the male body
Your J's contain something called xenobiotics, or a synthetic substance mimicking estrogen. By chronically puffing, you will accumulated these foreign "estrogens" and guess what happens to your body? The

same as consuming excess booze (gynecomastia boobs!) (4)

How come my body is less lean now?
Most of you guys were relatively active in high school with sports and other activities. This in addition to eating healthier at home helped you maintain your metabolism and leaner physique. As you know your college lifestyle is a bit different from high school, where you're not playing competitive sports and are in complete control of you diet. Any fat accumulated throughout the abdominal and waist areas is attributed mainly to poor dietary habits, consuming excess calories, and stress (insulin causing the body to store fat).

How does cellulite form?
Although more commonly hosted in the female body, cellulite certainly develops in the male body as well. The cells accumulate in the subcutaneous level and are arranged in chambers surrounded by connective tissue called *septae*. As water is retained, the fat becomes trapped within this area, expands and stretches, and eventually contracts and hardens (sclerosis), inhibiting flexibility of the skin. As the surrounding tissue continues to expand or weight and water gain continue, these areas of the skin continue to remain stagnant, while other sections bulge outward revealing cellulite (5).

Why do guys develop fat (and sometimes cellulite) around the love handles and belly?

The body hosts receptors that either break down fat (Beta-receptors) or create fat (Alpha-receptors). Above the waistline, the number of alpha to beta-receptors generally equates to a 1:1 ratio in both males and females. However below the waist, women have approximately 6 to 8 alpha-receptors for every beta (high cellulite region). This is the reason why women have difficulty losing weight in this area. Alpha-receptors (fat promoters) are generally stimulated by the consumption of carbohydrates, fats, amino acids, hormones, and alcohol (6).

Obviously the most effective way to eliminate the love handles, beer belly, potential cellulite, and overall weight gain.... is through a modified diet (chapters 4 & 5), exercise (in the next chapter... 8), and drinking ample amounts of water (remember ½ your weight; chapter 3). Of course cutting back on alcohol would certainly help.

Chapter 8

Your New Exercise Lifestyle
Introducing your 10 MINUTE TONE

This chapter teaches students: 1. The importance of exercise 2. Creating the motivation to exercise... extrinsic (which can be limiting or lead to stagnation) vs. beneficial intrinsic motivation 3. The three essentials to instill Motivation and promote an effective work outs (Mental Imagery, Workout buddies, and the Magic of Music all creating momentum) 4. The truth about your fat loss goals/Understanding how we burn fat through exercise (increased metabolism and through muscle enhancement) 5. How to tone abdominals effectively and why sit ups alone are ineffective for awesome abs/ The significance of the "Abdominal Vacuum" 6. The 10 MINUTE TONE TM (Beginning, Moderate and Advanced levels) 7. The Importance of stretching. The five most beneficial stretches to incorporate for post workout (Includes advice from expert trainer and Muscle Activation Specialist Ron Greenberg) 8. More effective exercise recommendations...and everyday strategies for burning more calories!

"If we all did the things we are capable of doing, we would literally astonish ourselves."

–Thomas Edison

Get back in front of that mirror again (just like you did in chapter 5 regarding the food choices you're making). This time ask yourself if you are satisfied with your physical appearance and decide whether you should include exercise into your collegiate lifestyle. If you

107

are satisfied with the way your body looks and don't care to change anything about it... fantastic! Congratulations! Must be nice.

Better yet, if you're a regular gym attendee or are presently conditioned to dart out for that morning run... excellent! You are far ahead of the game. Take a peek at the 10 Minute Tone any way. You may want to incorporate it into your workout routine. Remember knowledge is power!

Now, for those of you chronic loungers dissatisfied with your appearance, it's time to get off the couch (unless of course you're entertaining a guest), put down the playstation and make some basic lifestyle alterations. Time to MOVE... in the direction of achieving the weight loss/fat loss results you so desire.

The importance of exercise
Outside of getting in shape and reducing nasty hangover symptoms, exercise provides a multitude of health benefits that you will not only reap from now but far into the future. When we move or exert ourselves in anyway, oxygen flows to build muscle tissue and stronger bones. Since the heart is an actual muscle, when we exercise this organ, it too becomes strong and remains in a healthy state. Plus exercise is probably one of the best stress reducers on the market... and it's FREE!

Creating Motivation
One of the biggest problems people have with working out is not so much doing the actual exercises, but getting around or making the time to do it. Most people view working out as a chore that has to be squeezed into their day. After work people just want to go home, kick their feet up, and eat dinner. Getting on a treadmill isn't the most appealing idea after a long strenuous work day. Finishing midterms or completing a ten-page paper warrants party time not going to the gym. Students want play time after spending grueling hours in the library or listening and taking notes all day in lecture halls. Time is so precious to each and every one of us... This is the major reason for creating the Ten Minute Tone. It's fast, simple and effective. Better

yet, it requires no equipment, you can do it anywhere, and it doesn't cost a cent!

Extrinsic Motivators
As a trainer, the time I do see people most motivated to workout is usually before a big event: a wedding, a class reunion, going on a tropical vacation, and of course bathing suit weather (summer). "I have to lose 10 pounds before this wedding," or "I can't be looking like this in a bathing suit; especially in front of my boyfriend/girlfriend!" Notice something here? All of the motivation to exercise is for someone or something else, not you. What happens when the wedding is over or Labor Day finally green lights you to put your clothes back on? Is it back to late night ice cream and pizza? Don't get me wrong. It's great to see people working out at all. Just be careful… this type of motivational mindset can be limiting or cause you to revert back into stagnation (i.e. gaining the weight back).

Intrinsic Motivators
Now there's this racy girl who works out at the same gym where I presently train my clients. By observing the speed and air she catches soaring along on the treadmill, sometimes I thing she'd be an ideal candidate for the NFL. What makes her clock up there with a cheetah for 1+ hours and all the while hosting a look of either pure bliss or determination on her face? The girl literally enjoys just flying along on that machine either with earphones on or waving hello to everyone on staff. Better yet, she is so inspiring that I love to walk my clients by her launching pad just to provide them with a live illustration of pure internal motivation. "How does she find the energy?" clients ask.

This is an example of someone who works out for herself and not for someone or something else. She does it because she *wants to* and has embraced exercise as an important part of her life… she makes the time!

The Three Essentials that instill Motivation
How does a person learn to permanently adopt working out as part

of their daily routine? Outside of weddings and working off the pepperoni pizza from the night before "the guilt workout," there are three factors that I have found to really instill enjoyment and the commitment to exercise.

Mental Imagery

When you are exercising/working out, what are you thinking about? "Uggg when is this going to end?" or "I'm gonna ace that test! With these grades I know I can get into law school!" Listen to the difference. Who do you think is burning more calories during their workout? Uh definitely the future butt-kicking lawyer. Better yet this positive thinker is most likely associating their exhilarating thoughts with the exercise they're doing. This individual is most likely enjoying the exercise and will probably be committed to do it more often. Now you...think about positive things. Maybe it's the party you're psyched for on Friday night, or that "A" you just earned in Chemistry. If you're running, perhaps think about racing in a marathon and actually winning. Or fantasize about that hot guy/girl you just met. Dream away!

Workout Buddies

This is one of the fastest ways to get through a workout. Make sure you choose one who exerts physical effort and not just there to chit chat. It's amazing how effective group exercise/or working out in pairs can make burning calories fun and fly by. You can also teach each other new exercises, hence enhancing your workout even more!

Music

This is probably my favorite way to kick it into high gear. If you crank your favorite tunes; the ones that make you want to dance or move, this will bring magic into your workout. Better yet, you'll start associating your favorite songs with exercising. Plus, when you're jazzed up mentally, you will naturally workout harder and burn more calories.

Momentum

What happens when you develop that inner drive to exercise or to accomplish any goal for that matter? You've established an internal momentum! This is key for a successful workout and the three tips mentioned above create just that (mental imagery, a positive workout buddy, and your favorite music). Think of it this way... your favorite baseball team is down five runs in the eighth inning. Then out of nowhere they start playing out of their minds and come back swinging to win by two runs in the ninth! That's collective team momentum or that "invisible unseen movement."

The Truth About Your Fat Loss Goals

I know this topic can get annoying because every micromanaging boss or instructor makes you set them religiously already... outside of hockey and soccer, I agree. The topic frankly bugs me to the point where I have a client who literally refers to goal setting as limiting.... He's pretty right on. I'm just here to clarify your fat loss goal, okay? Ninety percent of the people I train have the same dream: the desire to lose fat. Whether it's around the waistline, in the hips/thighs, or upper arms... the same rules apply.

Losing fat is not a direct action (there is no such thing as fat spot reduction). We have a predetermined number of fat cells in the human body. The body reduces the size of those fat cells all over the entire body at various rates of speed, but it can't lose in just one area specifically. Let's say you have more fat cells in your hips than in your legs. You'll see a different rate of loss over time. The fat on your hips will take longer to dissipate.

Instead it is a reaction of three/four things: increasing your metabolism through proper diet (as we discussed in chapter 5), cardiovascular exercise and through muscle enhancement or strength training. Fortunately the Ten Minute Tone incorporates both cardiovascular and muscle building/strength training. What you put into your mouth is in your hands.

The Truth about ABS

This brings us to the topic of abdominals. There are countless products are out there.... Abs of steel, The Ab belt, Ab roller etc..

The majority are only gimmicks promising the ultimate six-pack. In addition, let it be known that 500 abdominal exercises a day aren't the secret to chiseled abs either. Isolated ab exercises are only about a quarter of the recipe for an awesome midsection.

It's a combination of cardiovascular activities, strength training, some direct abdominal exercises, and diet that play a part in whether you can have a flat stomach or host a six pack. To reveal a toned mid section, body fat levels simply need to drop.

Pulling your belly button towards your spine or "The abdominal vacuum" Do this during ALL exercises (including the Ten Minute Tone)! It works your Transverse Abdominis which is the muscle that holds your tummy tight. It activates your internal weight belt. Basically, it's a thin sheet of muscle running along the sides of the abs joining connective tissue, serving as your body's natural corset. Every time you suck in your stomach you are using this muscle. Do not hold your breath. Pull your abs in, and brace yourself as if someone were about to punch you in the stomach.

Avoiding low back pain
According to the Oregon Health and Science University, low back pain is one of the most significant health problems. They've obtained these statistics from the National Institute of Health (NIH):
Seventy to 85 percent of all people have back pain at some time in their life.

Back pain is the most frequent cause of activity limitation in people younger than 45 years old.

The following may help to prevent low back pain:
- practicing correct lifting techniques
- maintaining correct posture while sitting, standing, and sleeping
- exercising regularly (with proper stretching before participation)
- avoiding smoking

- maintaining a healthy weight
- reducing emotional stress which may cause muscle tension

The following exercises work to strengthen the muscle regions throughout the glutes, back, legs, and abdominals, hence promoting correct posture, the strengthening of core muscles, and reduction of overall body fat.

THE TEN MINUTE TONE

The beauty of the following workout is that you don't need any equipment at all; you're using your own body weight. As we discussed exercise and physical activity can extend our life, reduce the chances of being overweight; reduce stress, and wards off heart disease.

This exercise regimen isn't just for the freshmen 15… it's also perfect for eliminating the Sophomore seven, the junior juggle, and Senior Slouch. You upper classmen need to get up and move just as much as the new students. It's essential to develop and maintain proper workouts and healthy eating habits throughout your entire collegiate career. Statistics show that those students who tend to gain and accumulate weight throughout college have a higher likelihood of keeping it on into the post graduate years! So let's instill that positive lifestyle in you too. Better yet, you parents out there are just as capable of joining in. So here you go…

Start with 1 minute of Burpies: The name may sound funny, but trust me you won't be laughing after a minute of these exercises (that's why there are two levels to help ramp you up, beginner and advanced)… warning- these are a lot tougher than they seem! If there is one thing that will boost your heart rate and cause you to become winded this is it! I've had friends, colleagues, and student athletes in the best shape of their lives do just a one-minute set of these, and all of them were panting looking at their watches saying "No way Tim! That felt longer than a minute!" Showing them my watch I responded, "Yeah guys, like I control Father Time."

1. Bend down, 2. Place your hands on the floor (about shoulder

length apart), 3. Kick your feet back to where you're in a push-up position, 4. Jump your feet back to where your hands are (in between the hands) 5. Then jump straight up with your arms in the air.

Okay these are extremely challenging and exhausting so there are two levels:

Beginning: Do steps 1-4 (skip the jump at the end)

Advanced: Do steps 1-5 (add the jump at the end)

Alternatives

These are pretty tough to do and if you are not used to any exercise at all, they may be a bit too strenuous at first. So... (no you're not getting out of this first step... remember increasing your heart rate is key to weight loss) go ahead and substitute one minute of jumping jacks instead as a very beginning stage. Then as the jacks become too easy or ineffective for increasing your heart rate, do 30 seconds of burpies and 30 seconds of jacks, hence ramping your way up to solely doing burpies. Sound fair? No discouragement here!

30 seconds of push-ups

Push-ups are by far one of the best exercises you'll ever do for your upper body. Not only are you encompassing the muscles of the chest, shoulders, and triceps simultaneously, you are also working your core strength (glutes, hips, lower back, and YES ABS) and balance. This first round of push-ups should be done with the hands shoulder length apart and if this exercise is something you've never done before, than start out with a modified push-up off your knees and eventually progressing to doing them off your toes.

There are three levels of difficulty:

1: Off of the knees

2: Off of the toes

3: Off of the toes and add a Clap

Alternating lunges with rotation (1 minute)

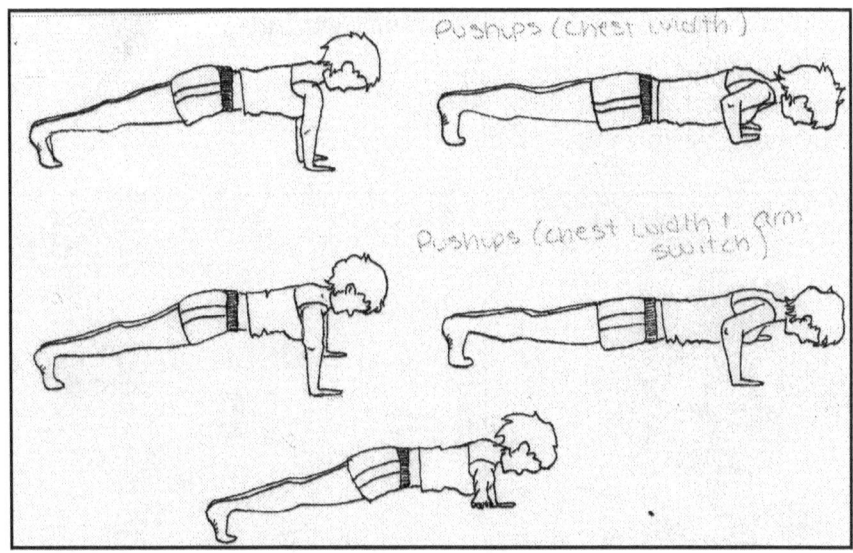

These types of lunges are extremely effective for working and toning almost every muscle in the body: Hips, Thighs, Glutes, Abs, Arms and back. Stand straight with your feet together. Hold both arms out in front with your hands together as if you were holding a gun (told you I loved Charles Angels growing up).

Step forward with the right leg and lower the left leg until the knee almost touches the floor. This lowered position is where you should focus on feeling the glutes contract.

Push off your right foot slowly returning to the starting position. Alternate the motion with the left leg to complete the set. Inhale while stepping forward and exhale while returning to the starting position. The step should be big enough that your left leg is nearly straight. Do not let your knee touch the floor. Make sure your head is up and your back is straight. Your chest should be lifted and your front leg should form a 90-degree angle at the bottom of the movement. Your right knee should not pass your right foot. You should be able to see your toes at all times.

The arm rotation: As your left leg lunges forward, while keeping the arms straight, move the hands around to the left side all the way

around to the side of the waist. For the right leg, move the extended hands around to the right.
Beginner: perform off of the knees
Advanced: perform off of the toes

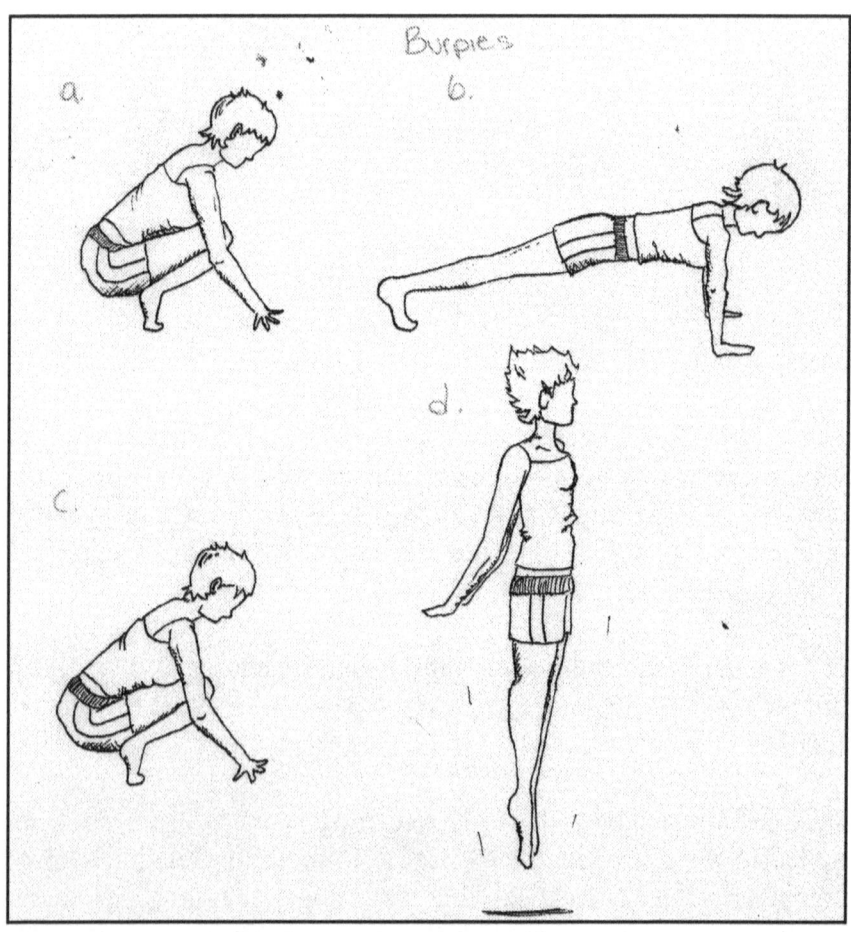

30 seconds of Triceps push-ups
This is the same as the push-ups mentioned above except you are going to place the hands closer together (one hand under each breast). These push-ups strengthen and define the tricep muscles (2/3 of the upper arm).

Three levels of difficulty

1. Do them off of the knees
2. Off of the toes
3. Add a clap at the end

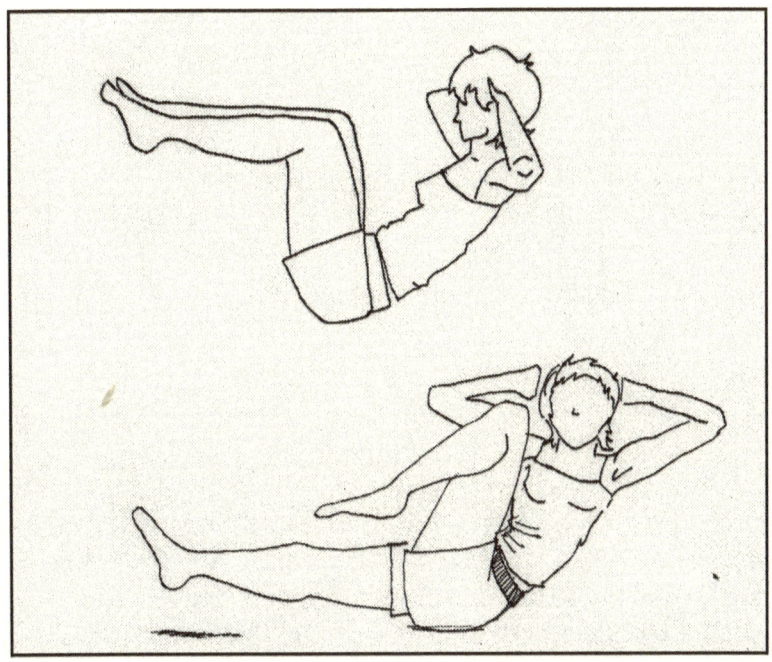

One minute of the Bicycle Abdominal maneuver The "Bicycle" still rates by researchers as one of the best abdominal exercises. It works all of the abdominal muscles at once… extremely effective. Begin by lying on the floor with your lower back in a neutral position. Loosely place your fingertips on either side of your head by your temples. Bring your knees up to about a 45-degree angle. Slowly go through a bicycle pedaling motion alternating your left elbow to your right knee, then your right elbow to your left knee.

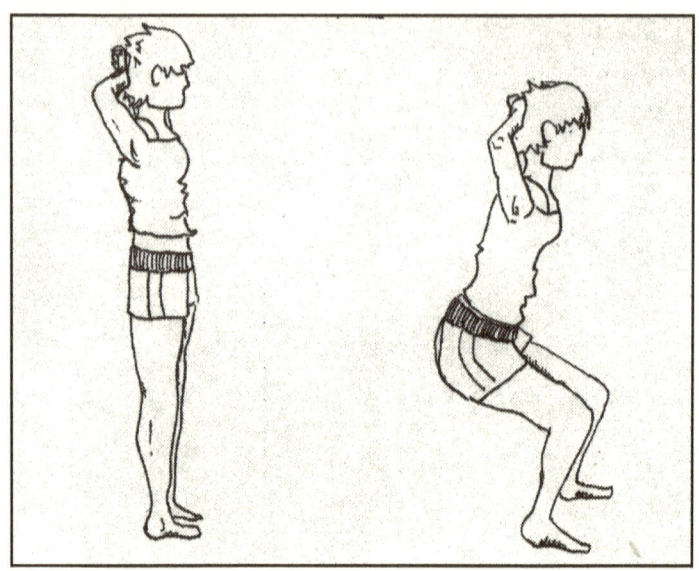

One Minute of Squats

I always say to clients that if you don't do squats as part of your lower body workout, than frankly you didn't have a 100% lower body workout. Squats work every muscle in your body from the waist down, as well as your abs and lower back. They certainly aren't as winding as your new burpie exercises, but you will certainly feel some form of a burn. Stand with your feet shoulder width apart, than lower your body down and back as if you were sitting in a chair. Then return to the standing position, and keep repeating. Don't let your knees ride excessively over your toes (it's best if you can see your feet at all times). Try to keep your back as close to the bed, stair, chair, etc... This is to ensure that you are working the arms and not the upper back. Now remember, the faster you do these the higher your heart rate will be (i.e. burning more calories). Now outside of speed, there are two levels to do squats:

Beginner: Just squat down and up

Advanced: Add a jump upon coming back up

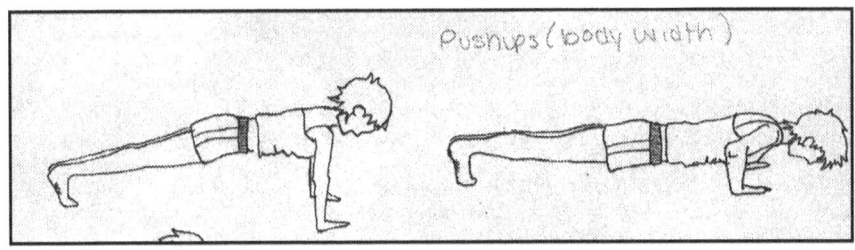

One minute of Push-ups with a rotation

The arms should be placed shoulder length apart like the first set. Lower yourself down and as you are pushing your body back up raise your left arm 180 degrees. Your head and rest of the upper body should rotate back with the straight arm. Then bring it back into the shoulder length position again. Lower yourself down and up again. As you come back up, do the same 180 degree rotation movement on the right side. Keep repeating and alternating for the full minute. The added rotation is excellent for strengthening and defining the back muscles.

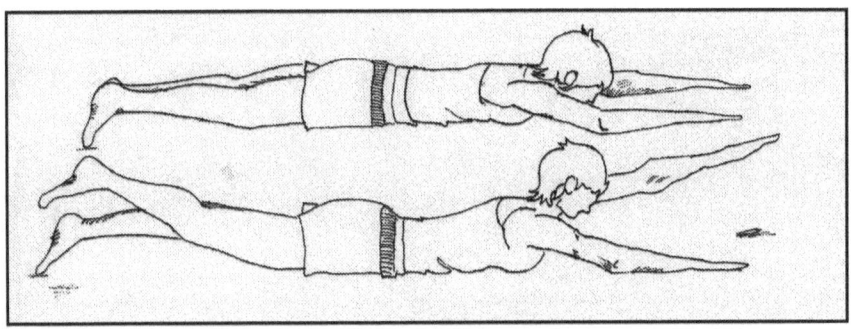

Low Back Extensions ("Supermans") one minute

No, don't go trying to fly off of your balcony like the super hero! It is also known as the "swan position" in Pilates. It is performed in a lying flat face down position with both arms straight out in front of you. As you raise your arms and upper body up, elevate the feet and legs at the same time. Hold this position for a few seconds and then keep repeating for the entire minute. This strengthens the glutes, along with the entire back core.

Beginner: only elevate the arms and upper body

Advanced: Elevate both the upper and lower body

Jump Lunges 30 seconds

Not quite as winding as burbies, but jump lunges will kick the heart rate back up. The difference between these and regular lunges is: You are switching/alternating legs in mid-air. So, get in lunge position (doesn't matter which leg you start with first). First, do a lunge, that when you come back up, jump up and switch the position of the legs. Then do another lunge and pop back up and alternate legs again. Keep repeating this for the entire 30 seconds. Whew! Great for the glutes, hips, thighs, abs, and core.

Beginner: Do 15 seconds of stationary (in place) lunges on each leg
Advanced: Perform the instructed jump lunges

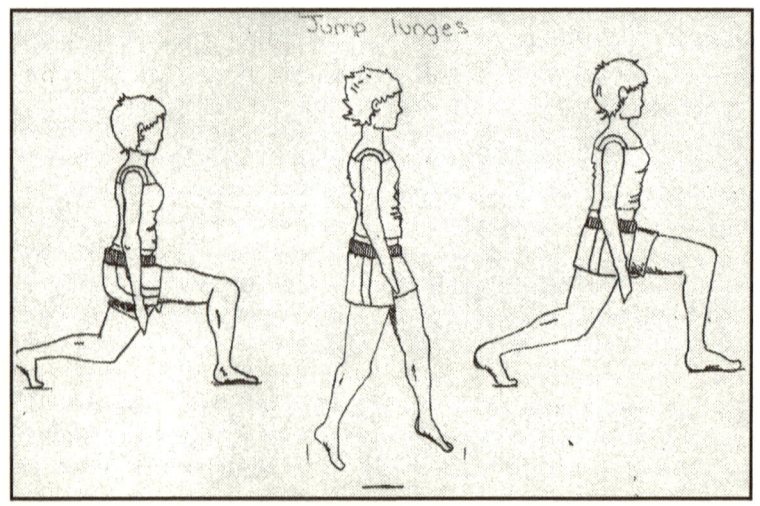

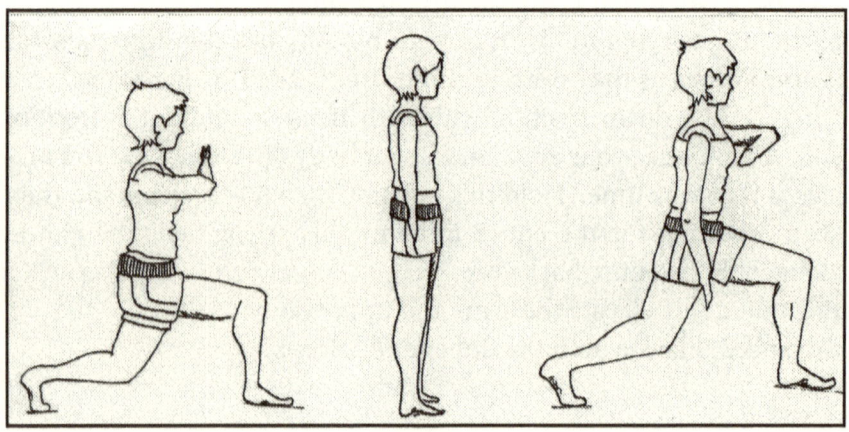

30 seconds of Dips

For this arm toning exercise you will only need a chair, a couch, a bed, or a stair. With your back facing the chair, couch etc., place your palms on the edge of the support ledge with your hands facing forward. Than just slowly lower your body with the weight on your hands and then slowly push yourself back up. And keep repeating down and up for the 30 seconds. Do not use the shoulders; the weight should be placed solely on the palms and back of the arms.

One more minute of burpies (or the modified jumping jack option)

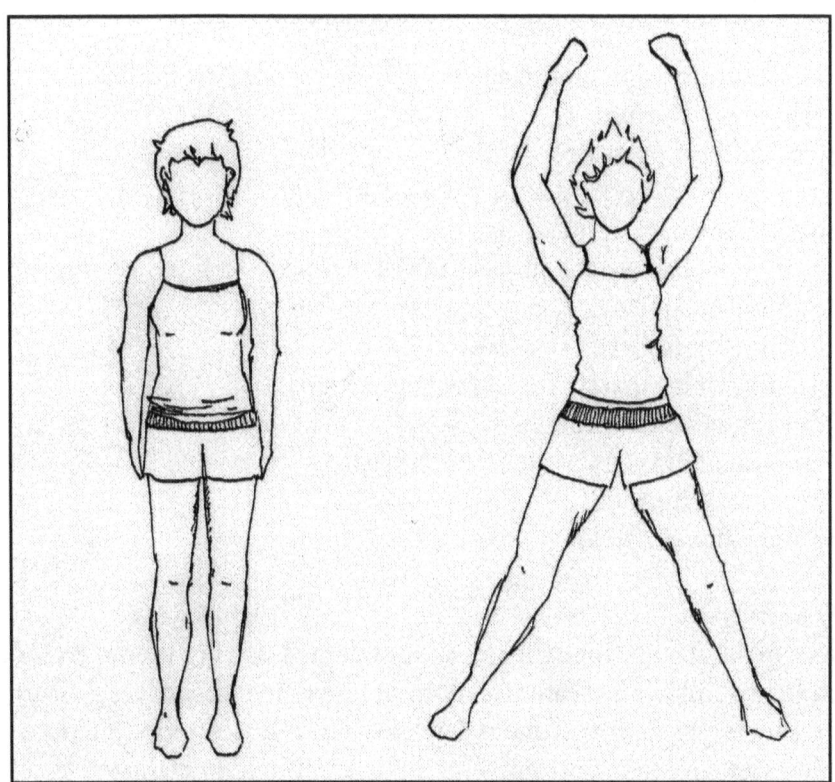

30 Second Plank Hold

Start by positioning your body face down on the ground: Get on your elbows having them face forward. Bring your knees off the ground and rise up onto your toes. Keep your entire body completely straight in perfect alignment (i.e. like a plank). Do not arch your back. Pull your abdominals up and your belly button towards your spine "The

Abdominal Vacuum." Hold this position for the entire 30 seconds. This helps to strengthen the entire core and abdominals.

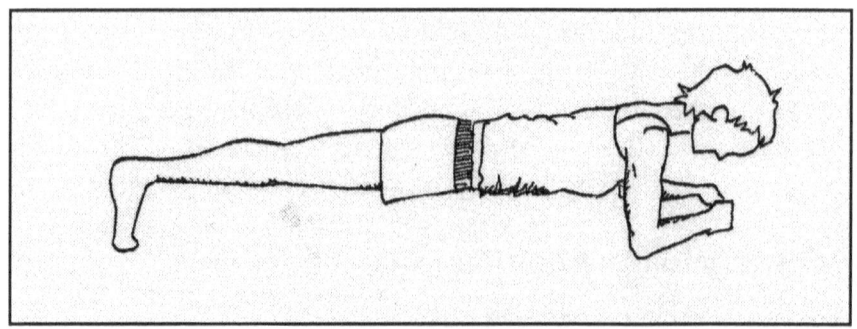

With of course any modifications, here's The Ten Minute Tone:
1 minute of Burpies
30 seconds of push-ups
1 minute of alternating lunges w/rotation
30 seconds of tricep push-ups
1 minute of bicycle abs (fingers to the temples)
1 minute of squats
1 minute of push-ups w/rotation
1 minute of low back extensions (supermans)
30 seconds of Jump lunges
1 minute of dips (use couch/bench/bed)
1 minute of Burbies
30 second plank hold

Stretching
As a general rule, once the muscle is warmed up (i.e. after exercise), stretching allows a greater freedom of movement, improves posture, promotes physical and mental relaxation, releases muscle tension, alleviates soreness, and prevents injuries. It is important to stretch after any exercises you choose.

Together with my colleague, Ron Greenberg an expert trainer and Muscle Activation Specialist, we have put together five safety stretches to perform post workout for non injured/pain free individuals and three to perform if you are feeling pain or strain in specific areas of the body.

The first five are traditionally recommended stretches by the National Academy of Sports Medicine (both Ron and I are certified in) and the five rehabilitating movements are derived from the modern technique of Muscle Activation Therapy…from which Ron is certified in and practices daily.

Remember a stretch should never hurt or be painful. By pulling on a muscle that is already sore or in pain, you are only doing it more damage. Instead, what you need to do is strengthen the muscle(s) surrounding or counterbalancing the overly tired or inhibited muscle. This in turn allows the muscle the time it needs to heal, or return into its regulated non inflamed state.

No Injuries/No Pain

Doorway stretch: For alleviating tightness in the chest area (pecs and anterior delts). This stretch is also beneficial for females who are larger breasted, for it may cause a lady to hunch over more. In a doorway, raise both arms up 90% on either side of the doorway. Lean forward and hold the stretch about 30 seconds

2. Hip-Flexor Stretch: These muscle groups are located directly above the thighs and right below the Transverse Abdominus (lower abs). They are connected to the pelvis, spine, upper fermers, and hip joints. Excessive tightening in the hip flexors may lead to lower back, glute, and even knee pain. Sitting in class or at a computer may cause the flexors to become tight or weak. Two ways to successfully stretch these muscles:

a: Get down on one knee and step the other out in front forward in a 90 degree angle with the front foot on the floor. Keep your posture as straight as possible. You should feel pull or a comfortable stretch in the flexor area. Switch legs and do the same thing on the other side.

b. Stand with one leg straight out and the other slightly back behind it (60 degree angle in between the legs. With the back leg, turn the foot in 10 degrees. Tilt the upper torso slightly back and you should feel a comfortable stretch in the hip flexor area. Switch legs and do the same with the other side.

3. Child's pose: So common in both yoga and Pilates today. Great! We all need to be doing this therapeutic stretch. It loosens tight lower, middle and upper back muscles that may be causing pain. Lay down with your legs (knees tucked) folded underneath you. Place your face down on the floor and arm straight out in front of you or by down by your sides. Hold this position for one minute. It feels great!

4. Calf stretch (off of stair or step): When the calves are tight, many other leg muscles become affected in a negative way: the knees, the quads, and the muscles that wrap under the foot… ouch! Stand on a stair or step and lower one of your heels down as far as it will go. Hold on to railings for support with both hands. As you lower your heel down, you should feel a slight pull along the back of the calf. Hold the stretch for 30 seconds and then switch feet and do the other calf for 30 seconds.

5. Neck stretch: Tight neck muscles caused by studying (computer or book). They can cause headaches and tension leading to lower back pain. This tension can lead to lower back pain.

a. For the back of the neck, lower your chin down towards the chest and with a hand add a push downward to enhance the stretch… hold for 20-30 seconds

b. Sides of the neck… for pain in the left side, take your left arm lower it and push it straight down. Simultaneously, bring the right arm over your head and gently pull the head towards the right. Hold the stretch for 20-30 seconds and then do the same stretch on the other side.

Okay in some pain either from exercise or sitting at a computer all day?

1. The Neck
Let's start with that pain in the neck you've been tolerating and treating with Advil for too long. First the back of the neck: Take your palm (doesn't matter which one) place it on your forehead and push the weight of your head into the palm of your hand for 5-6 seconds push gently and release. Do this three times. What this achieves is a strengthening (activating the dormant muscles in the neck region). This in turn will take the pressure off the aggravated muscle in the back of the neck

The sides of the neck (in pain). In the same time 5-6 seconds w/ three sets, start with right or left....If the left side is experiencing the pain, place your hand on the right side and push your weight into the palm of the right side. If the pain resides on the right side, place your palm on the left side applying pressure into the palm. This will activate the pain free side and force it to start pulling its weight, while allowing the opposite side to relax and heal.

2. Doorway Stretch
These were mentioned above to do especially after upper body exercises or slouching from enlarged breasts. This type of stretch is extremely therapeutic if your chest region is in any pain… instead of holding the arms upward at a 90 degree angle and pushing forward achieving a chest stretch, step in front of the doorway. Hold both arms outward and push the other direction (your arms back) into the doorway. This will strengthen the relevant back muscles to counterbalance the pain in the chest area. Again giving the area filled with pain a chance to rest and recover. 3 sets of 5-6 seconds.

3. If the Hip flexors (the psoas) are in pain, it may be an indicator that the rectus abdominus (section of abdominals) or hamstrings (back of the legs) are weak and require strengthening.
Pelvic lifts: Lay on your back with your knees bent in a 60 degree angle with your feet on the floor. Gently raise the core upward, squeeze the glutes and hold the position about 30 seconds. Lower

the core and raise it again for another 30 seconds. This works to strengthen hamstrings, glutes, and core.(1)

MORE EXERCISES
**Always drink water while working out... or any time as we have discussed throughout the book. For the purposes of weight loss, drinking water will position the liver to convert stored fat into energy!

Cardio – How much cardio should you do? The more you put into it, the more you get out of it. If you're on the treadmill walking for 20 minutes at 3.5, it's better than nothing. But if you run at a higher mph (miles per hour) 6.0 on up for forty five minutes, the results will be more to your liking. Which cardio equipment is best? You choose... Treadmills, stair steppers, elliptical machines, swimming etc... they're all fine. The point is, as long as you're getting that heart rate up, the results will follow. That's what is important. You have to become winded in order to burn calories faster! Don't forget to follow the proper nutritional recommendations in Chapters 4 & 5!

WEIGHT TRAINING

Dieting places a lot of stress. It forces the body to not only lose fat tissue, but muscle mass as well. In fact, when we're not eating, guess where the body pulls the nutrients/energy from first? Sorry not the fat (don't we all wish). Instead fasting breaks down the muscle tissue first. If you do nothing but cardio and never lift weights, you will lose muscle (also called skinny fat). So strength training is essential to maintain a toned physique.

Most women are concerned that they will bulk up if they work out with weights. Many women think that if they just look at a weight they'll immediately begin to bulk up and look like Arnold Schwarzenegger. Not true at all. Women just don't have enough testosterone (approximately 1/3 the amount of men do) to build huge amounts of muscle. Unless you're on steroids there is nothing to worry about. In fact, the more fat you lose and the more muscle you gain, the leaner and slimmer you'll look.

By the way, physiologically, there is no such thing as tone. A muscle can only do one of three things: grow, shrink or stay the same. Tone was marketed to help attract women to health clubs and to keep them from viewing exercise as a threat.

Crunches on the Physioball The physioball is a fantastic tool in the gym; especially for abs. Plus it adds an extra cushion to help support the back. Position yourself with your back on the ball. In order to avoid neck pain and to ensure the abs are doing the work (and not the neck), place your fingers on your temples or crossing your hands over your chest is an option as well. Do not place them behind your neck! Slowly and with control roll your back down over the ball. Then lift yourself back up achieving a strong abdominal contraction. Do this 10-12 times for three sets.

The Reverse Ab Curl This exercise isolates the lower abdominal region. Start by lying on your back with your hands straight down next to the hips. Pull the belly button to spine; raise your legs, and keep feet in line with the ceiling. Then, raise your hips off the floor until you can't raise them any further. Stop when you feel a full contraction of the abdominals and slowly return to the starting position. Repeat for 10-12 repetitions, do three sets.

The Double Crunch Similar to "bicycle abs" in the 10 Minute Tone, the double crunch isolates both the lower and upper region of the abdominals.

Lie on the floor face up and bend your knees until your legs are at a 45 degree angle with both feet on the floor. Place both hands crossed over your chest or place your fingertips on the side of your temples. Contracting your abdominals, raise your head and legs off the floor toward one another. Envision pulling the navel to the spine (as with all exercises) as you contract the entire core. Slowly lower both your shoulders and feet back to the floor. These are meant to done slowly and controlled.

STEP UPS

With the palms facing the side of the body, stand behind a six-to12-inch high step and keep your arms straight. (The height of the step should not exceed 90 degrees when the foot is placed up on the step). Upper thigh is almost parallel to the floor. The shoulders should be positioned downward and the chest pressed outward. With your hands towards the floor, keep your head tucked back, but not stuck out like a turtle. Step onto the middle of the step with your right foot and then lift your left knee high (to hip height). Make sure you place the weight of your heal onto the foot stepping up. Step down with your left foot, and then repeat on the right side. This is a great exercise for the entire lower body.

* WALKING LUNGES

Stand with your feet hip-width apart, palms in. Take a large step forward and lower your body so that your front knee lines up with your ankle. The back knee is almost touching the floor. Push off with your back foot and take a large step forward with your other foot. 90 degrees in both legs… walk lunge 20 steps on each side. Similar to the one minute of alternative lunges, this exercise tones the hips, glutes, abs, and lower back.

*If in the gym, add 5 or 8 pound weights and perform an arm curl every time you come up from each lunge.

Going to the Gym?

1. Pull-ups/Chin-ups on the machine

Outside push-ups and squats, pull-ups/chin-ups are my favorite exercises in the gym. Fortunately, most gyms have equipment that will allow you to do a chin-up/pull-up with as little or as much as your body weight can handle. This movement incorporates the muscles in your upper back (which collectively, are the largest muscles in the upper body), biceps, forearms, and core.

Show me a woman who can pull up at least 50% of her body weight for a set of 15, or a man who can pull up at least 75% of his bodyweight for a set of 15, and most likely they both will have above average physiques.

4. Rowing Machine

This machine is available in most gyms and is absolutely superb for strengthening the back muscles and creating impeccable posture. The exercise is excellent for alleviating and preventing lower back pain. …throughout their lives nine out of ten people will develop lower back pain (next to the common cold).

Be aware of hypoglycemia

Hypoglycemia, or low blood sugar, occurs when a person's blood sugar becomes too low causing the following symptoms; shaking, rapid heartbeat, sweating, impaired vision, weakness and headache. It is most common in diabetics taking medicine to lower their blood sugar; however anyone may experience these symptoms from time to time because of skipped meals or too much exercise. To prevent these reactions, try to establish regular meal times, consume foods higher in fiber, and eat a balance of complexed carbohydrates, fresh fruits and vegetables, lean proteins, and unsaturated fats throughout the day. If the symptoms continue… go to the health center.

More Ways to burn extra Calories
"Thats's what's great about the Tango. You get Tangled up? Than you just Tango on- Al Pacino, "Scent of a Woman"

1. Dance! One of the most fun and effective ways lose inches is to get out there and move
2. Unless of course you're injured always take the stairs instead of the elevator.
3. While you're sitting in lectures or in other sedentary positions

pull your abs in 30 seconds at a time. Try to do as many sets as you can … (Abdominal Vacuum)

4. Wash your car
5. Cleaning burns a lot of calories
6. Park your car further away to increase walking distance
7. Moving/helping a friend move
8. Power walk alone or with a buddy to class
9. Go for that morning jog (or whatever time you feel comfortable)
10. Go rollerblading, swim, bike ride, ski, raft, hike
11. Invest in some hilarious friends. Laughing is one of the best exercises you can do for the abs!
12. Include an exercise class for a one credit elective (walking for 55 minutes)
13. Push-up contests with friends
14. Intramural sports/activity clubs. To find one, ask around at gyms or local community centers. Keeping up with the crowd also means you'll be challenged to improve your skills. Ask about organized workouts and races offered by local track clubs. Play volleyball, basketball, softball, badminton, etc. or join a cycling club that hosts group rides.

Final Tip

Mix it up! Even the most dedicated exercisers occasionally get bored with their routine. Do the 10 Minute Tone one day with a group of friends. The next day do it alone. Incorporate some long walks/jogs with friends or alone. Listen to music. Join an intramural sport: … Avoid a stale exercise regimen…. Outside of a proper diet, enjoying your exercise time is one of the secrets and keys to optimal fitness!

CHAPTER 9

CASE STUDIES

<u>Laura's story</u>: A nineteen-year-old second semester freshman implements the dietary, academic, and exercise recommendations (Ten Minute Tone) to 1. Pull up her GPA and 2. Lose the 12 pounds she had accumulated thus so far in her dormitory life. <u>Tommy's story</u>: A 21 year old first semester senior living with friends in an off campus townhouse. He applies the grocery shopping guidelines, heeds Don's legal warnings, and jumpstarts his intramural career along with the Ten Minute Tone to 1. Stay out of trouble, 2. Shed those 8 extra pounds/the beer belly he earned from the first three years of school and to 3. Regain the energy levels he once had in high school!

"American Girl!"

–Tom Petty
Laura

A second semester freshman whose jeans were getting way too tight due to gaining 12 pounds over the past five months. Her first semester grades were not exactly noteworthy because she was overwhelmed with her 20 credit class load and a bit too distracted by the cute boys down on the 3rd floor of her dorm. She and her new girlfriends were constantly caught up and reporting in on the latest hot guys and who was hooking up with whom...

In high school all of her grades were A's and B's. Now it's 20 credits worth of one B, 3 C-'s, and her first D+... in Chemistry. She had failed to turn in a lab report on time. This was very upsetting for her because her pre-college plan was to eventually get into medical school, but with grades like that... forget it! Back in high school she was a member of student council for four consecutive years and never missed the honor roll. Laura was a stellar award winning soccer player, and earned the second singles tennis slot three years in a row. She was voted best female athlete her senior year.

At home her mom was not only an English teacher helping Laura by editing her papers, she was a great healthy cook. She knew how to portion size everything for her daughter and served the family balanced meals daily. Her dad was a successful engineer always available to help her with her math and science courses. She was always well behaved, didn't drink or smoke, she just had a fetish for chocolate. Since she was the only child, the pressure to succeed was high. Her parents groomed her to be a scholar like themselves and their dream was for their only child to become a doctor.

Her Dorm life Diet
When Laura moved into the dorms, she came with loaded Costco-sized canisters of M&M's, chocolate covered pretzels, Nacho Cheese Doritos, and cherry sodas. She and her roommate had a lot in common. Not only was she an equally talented high school athlete and scholar, she loved chocolate too. She met Laura half way with stocking the dorm room full of junk: Twix bars, cheese puffs, caramel covered popcorn, chocolate covered macadamia nuts (a sweet little souvenir from her Hawaiian summer vacation trip), and Mountain Dew galore!

The two went exploring the campus to find classes and of course places to use their meal plan cards. Traditional dorm cafeterias are known for keeping their college students healthy and energized with heavy pasta surprise dishes, mashed potatoes, and other like starchy carbs. Like any good chef, he/she has got to make it taste good, right? A lot of the time the potatoes and vegetables they had to choose from were loaded with butter and oil. Shiny, bright, and tasty!

Dinner
So when Laura went through the line, she thought the potatoes and

veggies would help balance out her chocolate eating and late night munching in the junk-filled dorm room.

Little did she know, the "healthy foods" she was choosing to eat hosted loads of hidden butter and fat. And this is before diving into the fettuccini Alfredo. Then they had to hit the ice cream sundae bar for desert… of course with chocolate sauce on top.

Breakfast
Laura just loved the waffle bar offered in the mornings. She'd load up with all the warm maple syrup and have a huge glass of orange juice with it. When ready for class, she'd pop a chewy chocolate granola bar for a snack after her three hour lab.

Lunch
She'd either get a mini pepperoni pizza from the on-campus Pizza Hut with an extra large coke, or grab a ham and cheddar cheese sandwich loaded with mayo and all the trimmings with a large Coke. Never Diet Coke.

Coffee study dates
Laura became a regular at the coffee houses meeting friends, classmates and lab partners for coffee and cramming…to the point where her 20 credit crazy schedule was sending her in there at least five days a week. Bet you can guess what type of coffee drink Laura and her roommate ordered…. Yep, the double whip cream hot chocolate mocha supreme with of course the chocolate shavings on top… Remember those are higher in fat and calories than most dinners. She was drinking these yummy beverages all the time 300+ calories each!

Caloric Reality
Between all these "coffee" drinks, waffle breakfasts, pizza, mayo and cheese filled sandwiches, tall glasses of orange juice, lard hidden dinners, sugary sodas, and junk in the dorm room… she was consuming an average 3,000 calories per day. And this is a non-drinker we're talking about here. She didn't think anything was wrong

with her eating habits because outside of the fluffy coffee drinks, in her perception her diet really hadn't changed that much. She was just so active in high school sports (singles tennis and soccer are heavy cardio workouts) that she burned all the fat and calories off. Plus her mom didn't hide a bunch of lard in the veggies and potatoes. Now the only exercise she's getting is just strolling through campus.

The New Start

So when Laura returned home for Christmas break, she was totally disgusted with her weight gain and beyond frustrated with her grades. She did not want to let her parents down by showing them her report card. Then on top of everything else, she had a mad crush on one of the guys down on the 3ʳᵈ floor who loved to date around. Eventually over a healthy dinner, she told her parents about her grades and they advised her to work with the school counselor in creating a more realistic class load for the upcoming semester. In tears, she went on to tell her parents about the weight gain and how all the guys were just big players at school.

That's when her mom handed her Fit Drunk & Smarter. She had heard about it through the high school English department where she worked and that it was a great book for both parents and college kids to read. "What? Come on Mom! I don't get drunk and you know I'm not a bad student… but I am getting fat so I will look at it a little," she said as she grabbed it and walked into her room. While lying on her bed she read the first chapter laughing hysterically, "Oh my God, this is totally me," she yelled. Laura could completely relate to the girl overloading her class schedule with a warning about the E.R. Then she flipped to chapter 5 and laughed even more. She was identifying her eating habits through this section and was figuring out how to alter some eating habits.

New Eating Strategy in the Cafeteria and Dorm Room

After reading a few sections of the book, not only did she call her roommate (who gained a solid ten pounds herself), but shared the book with some high school buddies while she was home. Her high school buds went and bought the book themselves, but the real heart to heart conversation transpired between she and her roommate at school. "We have got to change some things starting with our snack filled room," she said as they both laughed about their chocolate habits and chronic snacking in their room. Together over the phone they put together their new snack inventory:

-Fat-free pretzels
-light popcorn (they had a microwave in their room)
-baked lays and baked ruffles
-Fresh apples, oranges, mini carrots, and grapes (for the mini frig)
-Stock up on the tiny bottled waters instead of the sugary sodas
- Whole wheat crackers

On campus, she decided to skip the waffle bar for a while... saving it for a weekend treat. Instead, she ate the whole grain cereals with skim milk, bananas on top, and a tiny glass of orange juice. She added a glass of water to her breakfast meal and when she was off to class, she threw an apple and orange into her bag for snacks while leaving the high calorie chewy chocolate granola bar behind...

At lunch she elected to ditch the pizza for a while until the weight was off. Instead, she ate turkey breast sandwiches with only mustard while adding all the shrubs (lettuce, tomato, cucumber, bell peppers and sprouts). She ditched the cheese, mayo, and implemented bottled water.

Dinner was tricky so she tried the baked potato trick: Scooping out 1/3 of the insides while loading it up with salad bar goodies. Then she added just a tablespoon of dressing and pepper to season it up. The mashed potatoes were deleted from her diet as was the fettuccini Alfredo. She then put in a request to the chef in the back to serve steamed vegetables and more red marinara sauces for dinner... they complied and it was offered the next week. Plus she switched to iced tea (sugar free), water, or a Diet Coke for an occasional soda.

To The Coffee House
She had no idea of the caloric content and fat that was in her coffee

drinks. Wow she thought as she learned to just order coffee and add a packet of splenda and skim milk. Adding more flavor, she added cinnamon (aids to curb appetite) and just a teaspoon of chocolate powder on top. Perfect... still the great taste with practically 20 calories!

Picking the Racket Back Up/New physical elective

They also discussed how they needed to get more exercise so they both agreed to bring their rackets back from home and start playing over the weekends or whenever they had the time. When her roommate was unavailable, she would hit against the board in the rec center... both great exercise and stress relievers. Laura also added a 1 credit elective through the physical education department (Walking for 1 hour Tuesdays and Thursdays at 1:00 pm).

Ten Minute Tone

The kids in the dorm were raving about this condensed, simple yet effective new work-out! Laura was able to do the 1 minute burpies with the jump because her cardio status was still up there. Same with the jump lunges. However the push-ups were a bit of a challenge for her at first, so she started those three steps in the beginner stages. After about three months, Laura had mastered this workout just like soccer and tennis. She was performing the Ten Minute Tone at all advanced stages (with the claps at the end of push ups). She also didn't smoke or drink. Oh yeah... and she had lost 10 of the 12 pounds she had gained.

New Class Schedule

Upon returning to school after break, Laura made an appointment with her advisor in the premed department. They strategized while they revisited her previous fall 20 credit hectic nightmare. From there they collectively decided that she needed to retake the chemistry course this next semester while it was still fresh in her mind. At the same time, they decided to take some three credit courses (not four) that were less challenging and time consuming so she could earn an A in that chemistry class. Admissions and records will take an average of the D+ and the new A (hopefully) and that would bring the grade up to an acceptable B-. The advisor further recommended taking two classes over summer school (only a five week session) to get her caught up to speed and ready for the fall.

After the spring semester, Laura received a report card of one A in chemistry (pulling the average grade up to the B-), an A- in English 101, a B+ in history 101, another B+ in economics 201, and an A in her one credit walking elective. Over the summer she took the five week session and received an A in political science 201 and another A in Geography 101. By the time the fall semester started, Laura had pulled her GPA up to a 3.3 B+ average! Back on track doc!

The boys!
After reading both the boys and girls chapters, Laura understood boys a little bit more, where their heads were at, and how their goals are not to be in committed relationships, let alone finding a wife while attending college. This dispelled any small fractions of societal MRS. Degree programming she may have had. In fact, it empowered her to focus her attention more on her dream of getting into medical school. She dropped any resentment developed about her 3rd floor crush, where she and John (he now has a name) now meet for lunch in between classes. Laura's confidence has gone up so much that seniors are constantly asking her out now. Sure she picks and chooses, but always remembers her dream of becoming a doctor! YEA! Go Laura. Earn that MD girlfriend!

TOMMY

A 21 year old first semester Senior whose first three years of college really took a toll on his physique. He graduated in the top third of his high school class and lettered in three varsity sports. Although he was a conditioned athlete, Tommy elected to dedicate the majority of his time in completing his undergraduate education while discontinuing his pursuit of sports… and of course partying. He refused to join a gym because his budget was tight, plus he felt embarrassed about going because of his perception of how he looked. And he thought exercise would be too difficult now that he had picked up a smoking habit from the dorm two years back.

He entered college as a 6'0," 190 pound kid, ripped from head to toe who loved basketball more than beer. Over the course of three years, he only gained eight pounds but now looked completely different. A lot of the muscle he had accumulated from high school sports had dissipated and his waistline had grown from 31 to 36 inches.

Now living a quarter mile from campus in a townhouse complex with his two equally sedentary roommates who also hosted "beer bellies" that stuck out as far as… well let's just say that these boys could use some form of calisthenics. One cracking open a bag of ruffles to watch Saturday morning cartoons, the other finishing off last night's midnight delivery: a double cheese and sausage pizza. Then there's Tommy, jumping on the couch with his box of cherry pop tarts to lounge with them for the next three hours. This was their remedy for recovering from the five kegger party they hosted the night before. NICE.

Outside of his morning sugar high induced breakfast, he basically turned lazy and felt tired all the time. He would drink an occasional glass of water, but his beverage list was mainly Pepsi, margaritas, and beer. The above pretty much summed up his eating habits: pizza, potato chips, and sugary breakfast treats. Not one vegetable (sorry, the greasy chips are made from a potato) or a piece of real fruit existed in their little college bungalow. All junk food.

One of his roommates had received a Minor in Possession (MIP) charge from spring semester right before his 21st birthday and was paying his dad back monthly because the court costs were pretty steep. A cop spotted him holding a labeled beer beverage at party down the street. He had to get a job at the local bar and grill to earn extra money.

Another friend of theirs had just gotten arrested for a DUI charge driving home from the college pub, and was really hating life. Although he was 21, the charges were nasty ($2,000 fine, 60 hours of community service, six months of classes once per week, and he lost his driver's license for an entire year). He didn't hire a lawyer and tried to argue his way out of it by himself. For not following legal protocol, the judge gave him the maximum charges!

Over the summer Tommy received the <u>Fit Drunk & Smarter</u> book as a gift for his 21st birthday. Of course he laughed at the title, but dove right into the book during his life-guard shift (T-shirt on of course). Upon returning to college, he pondered about how he ate nothing but junk food, didn't exercise at all, and frankly got scared because he too had left that same pub and driven home over the BAC limit hundreds of times. He thought, "What if it was me that cop was waiting for outside at 1:00 AM?"

Okay, time to make some changes here. The first thing he thought was… "Whatever, a ten minute workout… Please, how easy. This is going to be a joke." He attempted the advanced level of the workout (i.e. Burpies with the jump) in front of his roommates! Tommy didn't last 20 second before he was so winded that he fell back onto his couch. Laughing hysterically at him, one of the other roommates tried it. He made it 35 seconds before panting and falling to the floor. Calling over to their third buddy, "Dude get over here… you have to try this. It's brutal!" Putting out his cigarette, he walked over and tried the maneuver with the jump. Same result… 25 seconds sent him running to the faucet for a glass of water.

As Tommy handed over the book to share with his pals, he took off in his car and headed to the drug store to buy the patch. He thought, "That's it! I'm quitting the cigs and I refuse to be out of shape any more. Wow and thank God I still even have a car and a license!" So, the first step of Tommy's revival was to quit smoking for good and never drink and drive again.

At the Grocery Store
After smearing that clear sticker to his concealed upper arm, he headed to the grocery store and grabbed a cart thinking, "Now what was that golden rule again? Oh yeah, first shop the perimeter of the

store. That's where all of the healthy foods are." He went right into the produce section and put fresh apples, oranges, grapes, bananas, and grapefruit into the cart. Next he grabbed a big sack of potatoes and put them in the new health boat. Time to make some baked potatoes and cut way back on the junky chips. For salads, he grabbed some Romaine lettuce, tomatoes, cucumbers, bell peppers, and carrots.

Then over at the deli, he picked up a pound of freshly sliced turkey breast and light reduced fat provolone cheese. Next he looked down and recognized the words "whole wheat" on the bread labels. So he added two loaves of authentic whole wheat bread to the cart. Next to the bread were hotdog and hamburger buns too. "Oh that's right we're tailgating for the game next weekend," he thought as he grabbed some whole wheat buns too.

Okay, over to the meat section… He remembered from the book to buy chicken breasts without the skin, ground *sirloin* for the hamburger meat, and lean cuts of steak (very little white ribbing). Much better choices than the fatty cheeseburgers and chicken wings they're used to eating. He thought, "Yes this stuff can get expensive, but now that I don't buy $5 packs of cigarettes every day, I definitely won't be owing any court fees, and will certainly save a lot of money by doing more walking and less driving, so I can afford to eat healthier."

"Time for the dairy section… One gallon of 1% milk (my roommates and I aren't quite ready for skim… too drastic) and 10 low sugar yogurts for $10. Good deal! What else for breakfast? Oh yeah eggs… we're going fly through these, better get two cartons. I remember only one or two yolks and the rest egg whites while cooking in the pans that have never been used. Oh yeah, and I need that Pam spay instead of butter. Cool I can make omelets with the bell peppers, onions, and the tomatoes.

"Now entering the aisle… This is where the C.R.A.P. is hidden. What else for breakfast? Two tins of Oatmeal and three boxes of healthful cereals (Special K, Total, and Kashi) should do it. So long pop tarts.

"What can we snack on? Turkey jerky, low fat pretzels, wheat thin crackers with hummus, light microwave popcorn, and tortilla chips (how cool, they have blue corn) and salsa instead of greasy potato chips and fatty cream dips. Speaking of dips, we need condiments for sandwiches and of course the BBQ: The salsa is great, here's the mustard, low fat mayonnaise, low fat salad dressings, and low sugar barbeque sauce. Hey and we can use spices instead of all the ketchup we eat," he said as the onion powder, garlic, and meat tenderizers flew into the cart...

The frozen section: "Okay those fresh vegetables were pretty expensive back in the produce section. I've got to save some money here. I'll buy the frozen ones (spinach, broccoli, mixed veggies, green beans). A few bags of these should be good for now.

Alright, now the water issue. One case of bottled water and oh great there's that faucet mount on sale... a lot easier to carry than another case of bottles. It will fit perfectly on the kitchen sink," as headed up to the check-out line. Great start Tommy!

Ok eating pizza in college is a must, but he realized you can give your body and arteries a fighting chance by altering the order a bit (holding the sausage, pepperoni, and by not doubling the cheese). Domino's thought they had the wrong address when they delivered the new bell pepper, mushroom, onion, extra sauce, and very light on the cheese new pizza order!

Intramural sports
He agreed that he did miss sports quite a bit, especially basketball. So, he and his roommates agreed to join a team playing every Thursday night. They had so much fun getting back into sports, that they signed up for indoor hockey and softball in the spring. They even started a ritual Friday late afternoon-slosh ball game at the park connected to their complex. Of course if there were any ball players drinking beer in the middle of the park, they were 21! If there were any underagers, they were totally informed about the cops! Boy did they love trying to bust up the Friday happy hour games, but the rule

was…. if you wanted to play, you had to have your ID on you (NOT FAKE) so the game wouldn't get busted up.

The Ten Minute Tone

This new workout was not only implemented every morning by all three roommates, it became the hot topic of their parties. They won a lot of money betting people they couldn't complete the *advanced* workout in 10 minutes on their first try. Tommy started on the beginner level with the jumping jacks and doing the pushups without the clap. After 2 months of the beginner level, he was ready for 30 seconds of advanced burpies mixed with 30 seconds of jumping jacks. After four months he was performing the full advanced level workout, lost six of the eight pounds, the muscle definition was being restored, and his waist had shrunk from 36 down to 33 inches. YEA! And with all of these basic lifestyle alterations, his energy levels were high again.

The Bar

Tommy and his friends all turned 21 and now know the cops are just waiting for them to get into their cars from about 9:00 P.M. on. No one drives at all. Walking home or taking cabs. Thanks Don! They've also cut way back on the tequila shots and no longer serve or drink jungle juice. This is not only for health and weight purposes, they didn't realize just how high their BAC levels were getting on the weekends. Far less passing out and definitely no more puking!

Now the Girlfriend

He had been dating a girl named Jenny off and on for about a year, and his two roommates referred to her as "the nag" because she wanted more of his time. After reading the advice from Barbara De Angeles, Tommy realized that she wasn't trying to take him away from his friends, but just wanted to be included more in his life. So he started inviting her over more to the Friday games and to his intramural events. He noticed that she actually got along with his friends quite well and frankly was a blast to hang out with once he stopped pushing her away.

CONCLUSION

Okay, a lot of foreign information to digest. I know... especially the spooky police section on arrests, MIP's, and felonies etc.... but hopefully this book has brought some valuable insight on how to excel during these fun yet challenging years. You've been fully informed on how to prioritize academics over playtime, and hopefully now have a clearer understanding of the opposite sex, hence alleviating some of the stressors associated with dating. Just trust that this "New Balanced" inner discipline will pay off not only during school, but for your post-collegiate years as well.

Chapter two has provided you with safety information not only to utilize during college, but for you to keep and carry with you throughout life. Definitely pass along this valuable piece (especially the B.A.C. chart and the legal advice provided by Mr. Ramsell) to all of your friends, family, and eventually to your own children.

"You are what you eat!" Wow, how true is that statement. Now that you aware of the foods that promote weight gain, weight loss and optimal health... apply it not just once in a while, but make these eating choices a part of your daily lifestyle. Healthful eating coupled with a consistent exercise regimen (including The Ten Minute Tone) will not only keep the weight off, it will ward off disease, prevent illness, give you energy, and frankly.... it will help you live a longer and more peaceful life!

-Warmest Regards
Tim Marsala

FOOTNOTES

Chapter 1

(1) Dr Suess, <u>Oh The Places You'll Go</u>, Random House New York, New York. 1990T.M. & Jacket Art by Dr. Suess Enterprises, L.P.

(2) Dr.Weil.com 3/17/2000 Dr. Andrew Weil M.D.

(3) Abboud Dr. Soo Kim and Jane Kim <u>Top of The Class</u> How Asian Parents Raise Achievers and How You Can Too. New York, New York, Berkley Books, 2006.

(4) Chopra Deepak <u>The Seven Spiritual Laws of Success</u> (New York, New York,Harmony books. 1998). Chap. 2.

Chapter 2

(1) The Life Extension foundation's <u>Disease Prevention and Treatment</u> Expanded Third Edition, Scientific Protocols That Integrate Mainstream and Alternative Medicine "Alcohol Induced Hangover Prevention" pgs. 22-23.

(2) Perricone, Nicolas M.D. <u>The Perricone Precription</u>, (New York, New York, Harper Collins Publishers, 2002), p. 21-22.

(3) Ibid., p. 19-20.

(4) <u>Disease Prevention and Treatment</u>, . P.22-23.

(5) <u>Ibid</u>., p. 22-23.

(6) Foster, Hellen. <u>Detox Solutions</u> 14 Plans To Detox Your Life. (London, Octopus Publishing Group Ltd. 2003). P. 11.

(7) "Male Hormone Modulation Therapy A Hormonal Attack on Aging <u>Disease   Prevention and Treatment</u>,. P. 431.

(8) Foster, p. 39.

(9) "Depression" <u>Disease Prevention and Treatment</u>,. P. 233.

(10) Foster, p. 8.

(11) Perricone, P. 71.

(12) Ramsell, Donald, J. Ramsell, Armamentos, and Klis, LLC.

(13) <u>Ibid</u>.

(14) <u>Ibid</u>._

(15) Chandra, Tanmoy M.D. Babar and Associates. 2006.

(16) University of Oklahoma Police Department. 2006.

(17) <u>Ibid</u>.

Chapter 3

(1) <u>Disease prevention and Treatment</u>,. P. 22-23

(2) <u>Ibid.</u>

(3) Foster,. p.78_

(4) Foster,. P.11.

(5) Ibid.

(6) Ibid.

(7) <u>Perricone</u>,. p.72.

(8) Carper, Jean, <u>Food Your Miracle Medicine</u>. (New York, New York, Harper_Collins Publishers, 1993.) p. 471.

(9) Balch, Phillis A. CNC, <u>Prescription For Nutritional Healing.</u> The A-Z Guide To Supplements (New York, New York, Warner Books, 1996), p. 67.

(10) Carper,. p. 472.

(11) Balch., p. 228.

(12) Carper,. P. 133,135.

(13) Carper,. P. 313-314.

(14) <u>Disease Prevention and Treatment</u>,. P. 23.

Chapter 4

(1) Lee, John R. M.D. with Virginia Hopkins What Your Doctor May Not Tell You About Menopause. The Breakthrough Book On Natural Progesterone. (New York, New York. Warner Books, 1996.). p. 103.
(2) Levine, Mel M.D. <u>A Mind At A Time</u>. (New York, New York. Simon & Shuster, 2002). Chapter 4.

(3) <u>Ibid</u>.

(4) Carper, Jean <u>Your Miracle Brain.</u> (New York, New York. Harper Collins Publishers, 2000). P. 10.

(5) <u>Disease Prevention and Treatment</u>,. P. 23.

(6) Your Miracle Brain,. P. 46.

(7) Bell, Rachel and Dr. Howard Peiper The A.D.D. and A.D.H.D. Diet A Comprehensive Look At Contributing Factors And Natural Treatments For Symptoms of Attention Deficit Disorder and Hyperactivity. (Markham, ON and Sheffield, MA.Safe Goods/New Century Publishing 2000) p. 43-45.

(8) Ibid.

(9) Bell,. Chap. 5.

(10) D'Elgin, Tershia What Should I Eat? A Complete Guide to The New Food Pyramid. (USA, Ballantine Books, 2005)., p. 17-18.

(11) Balch,. P. 75

(12) D'Elgin,. Chap. 2.

(13) D'Elgin,. Chap. 4.

(14) Your Miracle Brain,. P. 81, 209-211.

(15) Your Miracle Brain,. P. 195-210.

(16) Ibid.

(17) Your Miracle Brain,. P. 244-246.

(18) Your Miracle Brain,. P. 337.

(19) Your Miracle Brain,. P. 195-210.

(20) Your Miracle Brain,. P. 210.

(21) Jensen, Bernard,. Foods That Heal A Guide to Understanding

and Using the Power of Natural Foods. (New York, New York Avery, a member of Penguin Putnam, 1993),. P. 68.

(22) <u>Your Miracle Brain,</u>. P.286-289.

(23) Jensen,. P. 29-30.

(24) <u>Your Miracle Brain,</u>. P. 164.

(25) ediets.com.

(26) Jensen,. Preface.

(27) Bell,. P. chap. 5.

(28) Your Miracle Brain,. P. 32-33.

(29) Your Miracle Brain,. P. 27-29.

(30) Your Miracle Brain,. P. 31.

(31) Levine,. Chap. 4.

Chapter 5

(1) D'Elgin,. P. 39.

(2) D'Elgin,. Chap. 3.

(3) D'Elgin,. Chap. 4.

(4) <u>Ibid</u>.

(5) <u>Ibid</u>.

(6) D'Adamo, Peter J. with Catherine Whitney Eat Right 4 Your Type. (New York, New York, Putnam's Sons, 1996). P. 23-28.

(7) Sears, Barry Ph.D. with Bill Lawren. Enter The Zone (New York, New York, Harper Collins Publishers, 1995.) p. 14-18.

(8) D'Elgin,. P. 112-120.

(9) D'Elgin,. P. 122.

(10) Jensen,. P. 55-56.

(11) Carabu Coffee, Inc. print out of caloric/fat content 2006.

(12) Balch,. Chap 4.

Chapter 6

(1) McGraw, Phil Ph.D."What Do Those Women Have That You Don't" The Oprah Magazine Jan. 2006: p. 45.

(2) Marsala, Timothy J. "Please Girls… No More Super Models, Boys love curves" ChicagoScene.com Health and Beauty Link May 2002.

(3) "Hangover Helpers" WebMD.com Nov. 17, 2005.

(4) Disease Prevention and Treatment "Male Hormone Modulation Therapy A Hormonal Attack On Aging" p. 431.

(5) Schwartz, Erika M.D. The Hormone Solution Naturally Alleviate Symptoms of Hormone Imbalance From Adolescence Through Menopause (New York, New York, Warner Books, Inc. 2002). P. 31-33.

(6) "Hangover Helpers" WebMD.com Nov. 17, 2005.
(7) Schwartz,. Chap. 3.

(8) Lucille, Holly ND, RN "Estrogen Balance Is Key" Preventing Cancer in Women Is Key-With DIM <u>Ask The Doctor Answers To Your Health Questions.</u>

(9) Bissoon, Lionel, M.D., <u>www.mesotherapy.com</u>

(10) <u>Ibid.</u>

(11) <u>Ibid</u>.

Chapter 7

(1) Naber, Pamala c/o Dr. Leon Tcheupdjian, M.D. "Peter Pan.." <u>ChicagoScene.com</u> Health and Beauty Link Aug. 2002.

(2) De Angeles, Barbara Ph.D. <u>What Women Want Men To Know</u> The UltimateBook About Love, Sex, and Relationships For You-and The Man You Love (New York, New York, Hyperion, 2001) Chap 4.

(3) <u>Disease Prevention and Treatment,</u>. P. 431.

(4) Lee,. Chap. 5.

(5) Bissoon,. <u>Mesotherapy.com.</u>

(6) <u>Ibid</u>.

Chapter 8

(1) Greenberg, Ronald Muscle Activation Specialist and Expert Trainer (NASM National Academy of Sports Medicine) 2006.

GLOSSARY OF RELEVANT TERMS

Alcohol- A colorless volatile flammable liquid, C_2H_5OH, synthesized or obtained by fermentation of sugars and starches and widely used, either pure or denatured, as a solvent and in drugs, cleaning solutions, explosives, and intoxicating beverages. Also called *ethanol, ethyl alcohol, grain alcohol.* Intoxicating liquor containing alcohol.

Antioxidant- an enzyme or other organic substance, as vitamin E or beta carotene, that is capable of counteracting the damaging effects of oxidation in animal and human tissues.

Balance- mental steadiness or emotional stability; habit of calm behavior, judgment, etc; to have an equality or equivalence in weight, parts, etc.; be in equilibrium.

Blood Alcohol Content (B.A.C.)- Percentage of alcohol in the bloodstream. The legal driving limit for *all* states is below .08

Calorie Any of several approximately equal units of heat, each measured as the quantity of heat required to raise the temperature of 1 gram of water by 1°C from a standard initial temperature, especially from 3.98°C, 14.5°C, or 19.5°C, at 1 atmosphere pressure. Also called *gram calorie, small calorie.*

Carbohydrate- Any of a group of organic compounds that includes sugars, starches, celluloses, and gums and serves as a major energy source in the diet of animals. These compounds are produced by photosynthetic plants and contain only carbon, hydrogen, and oxygen, usually in the ratio 1:2:1.

Cellulite- A fatty deposit causing a dimpled or uneven appearance, as around the thighs and buttocks. A popular term for fat that is difficult to remove by dieting and that often has a dimpled appearance. There is no physiological difference between cellulite and ordinary fat.

Dehydration- Excessive loss of water from the body or from an organ or body part, as from illness or fluid deprivation.

Depression- **A** condition of general emotional dejection and withdrawal; sadness greater and more prolonged than that warranted by any objective reason.

Discipline- Training expected to produce a specific character or pattern of behavior, especially training that produces moral or mental improvement.

Exercise- bodily or mental exertion, esp. for the sake of training or improvement of health: activity; calisthenics, gymnastics. 2. EXERCISE, DRILL, PRACTICE refer to activities undertaken for training in some skill. EXERCISE is the most general term and may be either physical or mental:

Fat- animal tissue containing much of this substance; loose flesh; flabbiness: *to have rolls of fat around one's waist;.* having too much flabby tissue; corpulent; or obese

Fiber- the structural part of plants and plant products that consists of carbohydrates, as cellulose and pectin, that are wholly or partially indigestible and when eaten stimulate peristalsis in the intestine. Food containing a high amount of such carbohydrates, as whole grains, fruits, and vegetables.

Felony- an offense, as murder or burglary, of graver character than those called misdemeanors, esp. those commonly punished in the U.S. by imprisonment for more than a year.

Free Radicals- an atom or a group of atoms having lost at least one unpaired electron And participating in various reactions

Habit - An acquired behavior pattern regularly followed until it has become almost involuntary: 1. The habit of exercising daily or looking both ways before crossing the street 2.Daily bathing is an American habit a particular practice or custom 3.The habit of shaking hands is another example.

Hangover- the disagreeable physical aftereffects of drunkenness, such as a headache or stomach disorder, usually felt several hours after cessation of drinking.

Heart Rate- The number of heartbeats per unit of time, usually expressed as beats per minute.

Homesick-unhappy at being away and longing for familiar things or persons. Acutely longing for one's family or home. sad or depressed from a longing for home or family while away from them for a long time

Inflammation- A localized protective reaction of tissue to irritation, injury, or infection, characterized by pain, redness, swelling, and sometimes loss of function. 2. *Pathology*. redness, swelling, pain, tenderness, heat, and disturbed function of an area of the body, esp. as a reaction of tissues to injurious agents.

Insomnia- Inability to obtain sufficient sleep, esp. when chronic; difficulty in falling or staying asleep; sleeplessness.

Intoxication- to affect temporarily with diminished physical and mental control by means of alcoholic liquor, a drug, or another substance, esp. to excite or stupefy with liquor.

Liver- a large, reddish-brown, glandular organ located in the upper right side of the abdominal cavity, divided by fissures into five lobes and functioning in the secretion of bile and various metabolic processes

Misdemeanor- A criminal offense defined as less serious than a felony.

Momentum- A quantity expressing the motion of a body or system, equal to the product of the mass of a body and its velocity, and for a system equal to the vector sum of the products of mass and velocity of each particle in the system.

Muscle- a tissue composed of cells or fibers, the contraction of which produces movement in the body. An organ, composed of muscle tissue, that contracts to produce a particular movement

Nicotine- A colorless, poisonous alkaloid, $C_{10}H_{14}N_2$, derived from the tobacco plant and used as an insecticide. It is the substance in tobacco to which smokers can become addicted.

Protein- Any of a group of complex organic macromolecules that contain carbon, hydrogen, oxygen, nitrogen, and usually sulfur and are composed of one or more chains of amino acids. Proteins are fundamental components of all living cells and include many substances, such as enzymes, hormones, and antibodies, that are necessary for the proper functioning of an organism. They are essential in the diet of animals for the growth and repair of tissue and can be obtained from foods such as meat, fish, eggs, milk, and legumes.

Refined Grains (another form of "empty" calories): Refined means that close to if not all of the nutrients (vitamins, minerals, & fiber) have been removed from the food product either to enhance flavor or to increase shelf life. Examples include white flour, "non whole wheat" breads, bagels, pastas, tortillas, crackers, buns, and rolls. "White" rice is also categorized as refined as are most cereals. However manufacturers will "fortify" cereals, by adding iron, B-Vitamins, and bran to compensate for the refining process and to replenish some of the nutritional value

Tone- that state of the body or of an organ in which all its functions are performed with healthy vigor. Normal sensitivity to stimulation

Whole Grains- Whole means that the grain or food product is unaltered, or still hosts all of its nutritional value (fiber, vitamins and minerals). Whole grains are found in Oatmeal, popcorn, brown rice, and breads/pasta/rolls/tortillas/buns that have the word "whole" in product: i.e. "whole wheat bread" or "whole grain pasta." Many food labels will read "100% wheat bread." This can still means that the bread has been baked with "refined" wheat flour.